HANDBOOK FOR CARIBBEAN EARLY CHILDHOOD EDUCATION CAREGIVERS

HANDBOOK FOR CARIBBEAN EARLY CHILDHOOD EDUCATION CAREGIVERS

Rosamunde Renard

Laborie Community Education Centre (LABCEC)
National Association of Early Childhood Educators (NAECE)

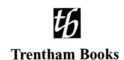

Trentham Books

First published in 1997 by Trentham Books Limited

Trentham Books Limited
Westview House
734 London Road
Oakhill
Stoke on Trent
Staffordshire
England ST4 5NP

British Cataloguing in Publication Data

A catalogue record for this book is available from the British Library
ISBN: 1 85856 102 7

Designed and typeset by Trentham Print Design Ltd., Chester and printed in Great Britain by The Cromwell Press Ltd., Wiltshire

Contents

Introduction

This handbook is designed for Caribbean early childhood education caregivers. It is based on work done in Saint Lucia by a community based organisation – the Laborie Community Education Centre (LABCEC) and a national non-governmental organisation – the National Association of Early Childhood Educators (NAECE).

LABCEC was initiated in October 1983 by me. It has helped to spawn at least nine other community based early childhood education projects in the south of Saint Lucia. Along with caregivers in the Castries basin – the capital of Saint Lucia – LABCEC was responsible for the formation of the NAECE in April 1996. The mission statement of both LABCEC and the NAECE is 'to stand up for the rights of children'.

In its fourteen years of operation, LABCEC has focused on developing quality early childhood education. This has included a parents-as-teachers programme based in homes as well as care and development in centres. NAECE is upscaling this work on a national basis.

I am 44 years of age, born in Guyana and a citizen of Saint Lucia. I am married with three children – two boys and one girl. I have a Masters in History from the University of the West Indies and am presently undertaking Doctoral studies in Education with the University of Liverpool. I was a secondary school teacher for 16 years. My life's main work has, however, focused on developing LABCEC and now working with other board members as a team to build NAECE.

Rosamunde Renard

Rosamunde Renard and Trentham Books would like to thank the German Embassy in London for their generous support of this publication.

Chapter 1

The advantages, benefits and characteristics of Community based Early Childhood Education Centres (CBECEs)

One of the advantages of CBECECs is that they can raise twenty to twenty five percent of their annual budgets through community funding. The Laborie Community Education Centre (LABCEC) is a living example. LABCEC is a small community based organisation (CBO) based in the village of Laborie, St. Lucia. Laborie has a population of only 1,304 persons according to the 1991 census. And yet in 1996-1997 LABCEC was able to raise EC $29,000.00 through community funding. This represents more than 25% of its annual budget and was raised, in order of priority, through local personal and corporate donors (EC$15,000*), rentals of building (EC$7,000) and photocopying services (EC$7,000).

Another advantage is that parents do not withdraw their children as much from the centres in moments of financial crisis. This is largely because of an in-depth continuing education programme furthered during group meetings. This can be proven by the fact that LABCEC has had a stable registration from 1985-1996. In contrast, two centres in the north of Saint Lucia which do not have regular parent meetings offering continuing education saw their registration fall from 60 to 34 and 24 to 12 because of a drop in the financial situation of the banana farmers. LABCEC caters for many parents who depend on banana farming too, but it did not witness this large decline in registration. BANCEC, another community based education centre linked to and supported by LABCEC, which is right in the heart of banana country, saw its registration fall far less severely: from 42 in 1995-1996 to 37 in 1996-1997.

* *Note*: EC$ – Eastern Caribbean Dollars – is the currency throughout this book.

1

CBECECs are also of benefit because they help to increase registration through continued education by making home visits to the poor and very poor. These home visits are made by local parent educators, prepared with the guidance of a manual adapted culturally and linguistically by LABCEC. The visits focus on education, including intellectual, social, emotional and motor development, in addition to health and nutrition. Through these visits poor and very poor parents become aware that early childhood education centres which are of quality are not simply child-minding centres but places where their children are well prepared for school and life. Some parents then make the financial sacrifice and send their children to pre-school – something they would not have done before. Such increases in registration because of this home visit programme to the poor and very poor have been witnessed in the districts of Laborie, Banse, Augier and Soufriere in Saint Lucia. In cases where the poor and very poor cannot make the financial sacrifice to send their children to the centres, they are now more confident and interested to help them at home.

CBECECs can also access funding from funding agencies. Most funding agencies request that centres be not only community run but also community owned. The few funding agencies which do not require community ownership require at least that the centres be community run. Over 12 years as a community based organisation, LABCEC has been able to access almost half a million US dollars for itself and other CBECECS, partly on grounds of being a community owned and managed centre.

Besides the financial advantages, there are profound moral and spiritual benefits. CBECECs help develop a sense of reciprocal responsibility. They foster the spirit that we are all responsible for one another. One example can be taken again from LABCEC. In 1994 LABCEC lost its recurrent funding from the Ministry of Community Development of EC$5,000.00 per year. Three of LABCEC's board members are also on the executive of the Laborie Credit Union. The Laborie Credit Union was approached to replace this funding. The three board members were solicited to help in the realisation of this request. In 1995 the Laborie Credit Union decided to give EC$3,000.00 to LABCEC annually. This is just one of the many examples of the development of a sense of reciprocal responsibility through CBECECS.

CBECECs also provide rallying points for social and political actions that build consensus and solidarity. The majority of people are very concerned about their children. Despite racial, national and other divisions, they are prepared to unite around the theme of their children. Because of their deep concern for their children, actions around these children help to foster consensus and solidarity.

CBECECs can heighten government advocacy. This is especially the case when they form networks or national associations. LABCEC is now able to access

EC$30,000.00 per year from the government for itself and related centres. Through discussions, documents and public support, the National Association of Early Childhood Educators (NAECE) is now encouraging government to increase its budget on early childhood education from the present less than 1 percent of its budget for the Ministry of Education and the Ministry of Community Development combined.

CBECECs influence not only government structures but also corporate structures. NAECE, as an organisation committed to promoting community based early childhood education, although it caters in different degrees to all centres, has begun to influence corporate structures. Between September 1996 and June 1997, it has raised EC$7,000.00 from the private sector. It is true that this is not much especially compared to the EC$16,000.00 it has raised from personal donors since that same date. However, it is a beginning which, if there is continued follow up, can be at least quadrupled.

Centres which are community based rely upon and build a knowledge base on early childhood education. CBECECs have twice termly parent meetings, at which education is an engrained component. CBECECs also have monthly home visits, when funding can be acquired, in which relevant and up-to-date education is also integral.

Democracy is promoted and authoritarianism restrained through CBECECS. For example, 80% of all Saint Lucians believe that beating children should be a main form of punishment. After parent and community discussions through CBECECS, only 20% of the parents and community who took part in the home visits, group meetings and discussions still believed that beating children should be a principal form of punishment.

CBECECs permit the community to negotiate with the larger society. For instance, at the start, many community members thought that all the children at LABCEC did was play. Through discussions with board members, staff, volunteers, parents and the wider community, the larger society came to accept that play was an integral part of children's learning.

Civic participation is encouraged by CBECECs. Of LABCEC's fourteen workers, eight are volunteers and do not receive a salary but only a tiny re-imbursement of expenses and a daily meal. They are indispensable to the quality of the centre: they provide quality care through ongoing training and, in addition, they ensure that there is a low ratio of children to adults. It is important to state that this is not a case of exploitation of the poor, because 90% of these volunteers are themselves poor or very poor. The volunteers have been for the most part unemployed for years and have little possibility of finding jobs. Some of them are young but choose to volunteer at LABCEC for a while. That they are shown love and respect is essential if they are to continue to give their quality time. A few volunteers come from higher earning socio-economic brackets. They work as fund-raisers and will serve as community based organisers. Civic participation is just as important in sharing ideas.

CBECECs are also constructive of community. They help to foster links among community members and organisations.

Finally, and briefly, these are the characteristics of CBECECs:

CBECECs involve all stakeholders: the children, parents, staff members, volunteers, board members, government and members of the larger community including other community based organisations. The community owns the centre. It is part of its financial patrimony. The community also manages the centre. Stakeholders or participants mentioned above meet in regular fora where they make policy and express their opinions. The board is the final authority and is composed of at least three parents, Principals of the local Infant and Primary Schools, a representative of government and a representative of the private sector. Also on board are some persons who are poor or very poor.

With the participation of all these different stakeholders, CBECECs are adversarial and conflictual. For example, many parents all over Saint Lucia think it is important for their children to learn to write their own names at pre-school. This is particularly so in Saint Lucia, with its relatively high level of illiteracy in the Caribbean. Some stakeholders are adamant – children should not be learning to write their names in pre-school. LABCEC, however, like all the CBECECs centres did not start from the view that the parents' wishes should be ignored when they did not fit professional tenets. Rather, much education was done on the importance of the pre-writing activities while attempts were made to teach those children at the centre who were ready, to write their names. Some participants of the CBECECs, therefore, need the skill to manage disagreements constructively, even if a change for the better takes years in coming.

The benefits of CBECECs indicate that *only* these types of centres can ensure quality early child care in the developing world and among underprivileged sectors of the developed world. Parents and government combined cannot provide enough resources to provide high quality centres. Early childhood education centres in these areas have to depend on the privileged sectors of the community for finance and advocacy and on the poor sectors of the community for human resources. To be able to do this, the centres must educate these stakeholders and involve them meaningfully. Without their education and meaningful involvement, these stakeholders would be unwilling and inadequately equipped to contribute the resources essential for quality.

Chapter 2

A case for community based Early Childhood Education Centres

Introduction

This section is dedicated to the pre-school and daycare administrators who yearn to help manage a permanent institution which is financially sustainable, to provide a service of high quality that will remain so for generations to come, and to earn a reasonable wage for all months of the year, and which most parents can afford.

It is also dedicated to the initiators in a local community – initiators who share the desire to have a sustainable, quality early childhood education centre with maximum participation of the community.

The booklet describes and advocates the establishment of small local institutions which are:

- community-managed: run by local boards, parents, staff and a wider membership

- community-owned: belonging physically and otherwise to the children, board, parents, staff and membership in the local community

- concerned with quality: meeting the licensing requirements of the local authorities and the accreditation criteria of relevant institutions

- financially, socially and intellectually sustainable: chiefly because trained, experienced and dedicated community volunteers animate and serve the organisation.

This chapter is based largely on the experience of the Laborie Community Education Centre (LABCEC) in Saint Lucia. Accordingly, it describes more specifically the structure and operations of that Centre, but in a way which allows this relatively unique experiment to be used and adapted to other situations and contexts. It is, therefore, hoped that this publication will assist others in their efforts towards the creation and management of community-run pre-schools and daycare Centres.

The Institution

The institution provides a pre-school and daycare Centre. It should serve children from birth to five years. Its programmes concentrate on:

1. pre-school and daycare catering for children from birth to five years. This centre should have an integrated programme of education, health and nutrition, including a food programme where possible

2. A Parents as Teachers(PAT) programme catering for parents and children, with specific emphasis on parents whose children are disadvantaged either cognitively, socially or emotionally.

For elements of a quality pre-school and daycare programme please go to Appendix 7 for questionnaire. I would advise you to do your own self study, allocating three marks for very much, two marks for sometimes and one mark for not at all. In each section a percentage of 95% or more means that there is very little room for improvement, 80-94% is excellent, 70-80% is good, while there is much room for improvement in each area where you score less than 70%.

Information about the PAT programme is provided below. Please write to LABCEC or NAECE at Laborie Post Office, Saint Lucia for further details.

The institution may also possibly include a food programme. No Early Childhood Education administrator should set one up without a minimum of fifty parents prepared to register for it. If the programme is low-cost, profits will be non-existent or minimal. So the motive for initiating a food programme will not be financial; it will be because parents have expressed a need for it. It should be made clear to the parents from the outset that the programme should not be viewed as replacing adequate home nutrition but only as supplementing it. Parents, however, do need some centres where they can drop off their children in the morning without having to prepare lunch and snacks for them. For a Director or Administrator to accommodate this need, certain obvious facilities are required, such as a stove, fridge, freezer, kitchen equipment, cupboards. The kitchen area should be clean and possibly tiled. Where a food programme is provided there will be greater empathy and cooperation between staff and children, who will feel more cared for and loved. Where such a service cannot be provided, parents must be educated on the importance of good nutrition for their children and on what foods to provide.

Not all parents can afford the cost of education, much less education accompanied with a food programme. Early childhood education centres should have a scholarship programme to cater for poor parents. Boards should peruse their budgets to see how many children they can reasonably give scholarships to – and do so. This caters for a need and helps to affirm that the Early Childhood Education Centres are run at low cost and by a community that genuinely cares.

A workshop should be held, in which the mission of the early childhood education centre is defined by board members and general membership. It is useful to have the workshop led by a resource person with experience in defining missions of similar organisations.

An early childhood education centre should be a caring institution, concerned with the interests of poor children and their parents. It should have a high degree of community participation in all its aspects. Quality should be striven for and the achievement of this quality necessitates the formation and follow-up of an educated, committed membership. All this should be taken into consideration when drawing up the Mission Statement.

Parental involvement

Almost all early childhood education programmes which do not have the involvement of parents have failed to sustain the considerable cognitive gains made by the children. Biber affirms that 'to work with children alone is to invite failure and frustration'.[1]

The period of most rapid intellectual growth occurs from birth to age eight. This is the age when children spend most of their time in the home environment. There are three alternative scenarios for the children. Either nothing is done for them, or they attend a quality early childhood education centre, or the parents are guided and supported in providing an enriched home environment and experiences for their children. Obviously, the first makes little sense. So it is to the second two that we turn, beginning with the third alternative.

White and Watts have noted that:

> Most women are capable of doing a fine job with their one to three year old children. Our study has convinced us that a mother need not necessarily have even a high school diploma, let alone a college education. Nor does she need to have very substantial economic assets. In addition, it is clear that a good job can be accomplished without a father in the home. In all these statements we see considerable hope for future generations.[2]

White further states:

Indeed, we came to believe that the informal education that families provide for their children *makes more of an impact on a child's total educational development than then formal educational system.* If a family does its job well, the professional can then provide effective training. If not, there may be little the professional can do to save the child from mediocrity.[3]

Juvenile delinquency, teenage pregnancy, indiscipline, school failure and persistent poverty have all created severe problems in Saint Lucia for generations. Recent reports have suggested that these problems are becoming more and more acute. It is evident that traditional measures have not been able to curb these rising tendencies. There is need for a community development strategy geared to promoting attentive parenting and healthy development of children. This strategy should not be confused with more superficial efforts to provide parent education by organising speakers for parents of young children to listen to once or twice a term. There is need for a parenting education programme which provides sustained education and support. This is particularly urgent for at-risk and special children and their families.

Parents need a holistic approach which is easy and attractive and so will encourage their participation. Parents need empowerment so that they understand and will try to play an active role in their children's education. The country's economic viability and the training of the next generation for work deserve as much support as they can actively get and Parenting Education is one sure measure of giving such aid through family oriented strategies. Research suggests that:

> Programmes that work with parents to strengthen parenting skills and to enhance familial and community context for human development can produce long term gains for children and youth in areas that are of particular interest to policy makers. Various forms of intra- and extra-familial social support can mediate parenting attitudes and behaviours thereby contributing positively to human development.[4]

Mothers complain of being overworked. They do not have enough time to spend with their children. Quite often, if the situation is examined carefully, time *can* be found. However, these mothers need to be encouraged to make spending enough quality time with their children a priority, so that their children develop socially, physically, intellectually, creatively, emotionally and spiritually. Some parents who are under-educated and possibly illiterate might not easily recognise the need to spend quality time with their children on their own initiative. In such matters they need education. This education is, as noted by White, within the grasp of even the illiterate mothers, precisely because of the age range of the children. Many parents of at-risk children have financial problems. They need the help and support such a programme can offer. Even small items like crayons, paper and other educational materials necessary for the proper education of their children may be a burden for parents. They need easy access to materials such as books. They also need to be made aware of the relative ease with which home-made and natural materials can be used. The parenting programme can provide such easy access and education, in addition to help and financial support.

There are certain patterns and beliefs that are a consequence of the Caribbean's history of slavery, colonialism and post-colonialism. One such prevailing belief is that physical punishment is essential for discipline. While it is not suggested here that a smack or two will hurt a child, the prevalence of sometimes extreme physical punishment is disturbing. Another disturbing historical pattern is the absence of men in family life as husbands or life partners. Where men are present, their habit of having multiple partners, of not playing with their children and so on can cause severe emotional traumas to mothers and their children. There is a great need for men to become better parents. The parenting programme can address this serious concern.

The objectives of this parenting programme, here called Parents as Teachers (PAT), are as follows:

- to curb the problem of child illiteracy

- to help children succeed in school

- to reduce failure in school

- to help parents acquire the basic knowledge, understanding and skills to enable them to adopt acceptable child rearing practices

- to help parents achieve an enhanced measure of self-assurance and respect, demonstrated through their increased involvement in a variety of activities relevant to their child's education

- to enlist parental cooperation in solving school and/or centre related problems, for example, discipline,

- to encourage parental participation and follow-up of their children's emotional and cognitive development up to   adulthood

- to help curb child abuse and other mental health problems related to children

- To aid in the alleviation of a mounting number of family related social problems such as teenage pregnancy, increase in juvenile crime, and inter-generational poverty.

The activities of this Parents as Teachers Programme include:

- monthly group meetings with parents

- monthly private home visits to parents and their children by trained parent educators

- the creation of a referral network that can help parents find special services that are beyond the scope of the parenting programme

- the use of parents as volunteers

- the participation of parents in the decision-making process.

Parents' Meetings

It is important to stress from the outset that while parent meetings can be used as part of the parent involvement process, they should not be the total programme.

Rationales for parental involvement in meetings include the following:

- to give parents a feeling of importance and support in their role as parents and educators

- to enhance the self-image and performance achievement of the child

- To change parents' attitudes about the school. This is particularly important where the parent has a negative attitude toward the school. It also helps where the parent has little knowledge of the school or its programme, for as parental knowledge about school programmes increases, parental approval of the school's programmes also usually increases

- to provide parents with skills they can use at home with their children

- to provide opportunities for parents to share experiences and form support networks

- to address parents' questions and concerns as they arise.

Making Parents feel Welcome

Some teachers are hostile towards parents. They consider them a bother and sometimes make them feel very unwelcome. According to Morrison, 'traditionally, schools have not been anxious to involve parents in the schooling process'.[5] Administrators have been heard to say that 'the parents are lying'. When parents make a report some teachers become very upset and what is worse, sometimes take it out on the children. All teachers should remember that every parent wants to be a good parent. They do not complain for the sake of complaining but because they are anxious about the quality of care and schooling their children receive. Early childhood education professionals should treat parents with kindness, love and patience. When parents make a complaint, they should be listened to patiently and the complaint taken seriously. Complaints should be discussed in staff meetings and the staff should not be angry with the parent for bringing up a problem. A decision should be taken regarding every complaint and this decision conveyed to the parent as gently as possible. On no account should revenge or hostility be expressed to parents, or to their children, because of criticisms made. Rather, criticisms should be encouraged because they signal avenues for improvement in the quality of the services rendered.

During parent meetings, time should always be left for parents' questions and concerns. These should be followed up at staff meetings and board meetings and at least two meetings after; decisions regarding the particular question or concern should be conveyed to the parents. Follow-up is vital; without it the parents will not take the institution seriously and, more often than not, withdraw their involvement, if not their children from the school, if the matter is serious.

Agenda for group meetings

The following is a sample of an agenda. It can be modified to suit specific situations. However, it contains the items which need to be covered in almost all cases.

1. Welcome

2. Sign-in sheet. This is very important as it is possible to gauge the level of parent involvement from centre to centre and to compare them. Where involvement is low, strategies should be used to increase involvement. A register, in alphabetical order, should be prepared with signs indicating those present or absent on each date; parents chronically absent should be contacted. Parents consistently present should be rewarded

3. Announcements and warm-up activities based on some activities done with the children

4. Introduction of speaker and topic

5. Discussion

6. Parents' questions and concerns

7. Evaluation of meeting

8. Any other business

9. Social time for the parents (if appropriate)

10. End meeting. Date of next meeting. In consideration of parents, limit the meeting to a maximum of one hour and a half.

Raising attendance at parents' meetings

Attendance below 40%-50% should be considered low. Even if attendance is 60%, efforts should still be made to improve it. A minority of parents, some of whom hated school, may never attend meetings despite persistent appeals. However, most can be persuaded to put in an appearance, even if irregularly.

One way to increase attendance is by visiting the parent at least once a year, preferably after three unattended meetings. The parent should know what was discussed and be encouraged to attend meetings. Each member of staff should receive his or her quota of parents and visit those who do not attend meetings at least once a year.

If after or even before a home visit, parents still do not attend meetings, then a letter should be sent asking them to come to the school on a matter of importance to their children. When parents come in they should be reminded about the importance and value of parent involvement through group meetings, and this should also be stressed in the home visits. Parents should be shown the attendance register for parents' meetings and where their names figure on it.

At the end of the year, each parent should receive a letter stating how many meetings they attended out of the total number held that year. If their attendance is high, they should be commended. If it is low they should be encouraged to come next time.

Parent meetings should also serve as support groups which help parents with social, emotional or financial needs.

Inviting Guest Speakers

Administrators must remember that guest speakers should be invited at least one month in advance, first orally to confirm the topic and that they agree to be guest speaker.

This oral invitation should be followed up – no more than one week later – by a written invitation. It makes no difference whether this invitation is typed or handwritten.

This written invitation should be followed up by a letter or reminder at least one week before the guest speaker is due to appear.

Finally, the day before, guest speakers should be reminded by telephone call or, if they have no telephone, the administrator should send a message via a neighbour or close relative.

It is important, also, to remember that guest speakers are there not only to educate but to be educated. For each topic that guest speakers are asked to talk about – even if they are specialists on the topic – the centre must provide them with research material. The Administrator should also ask guest speakers for a written copy of their speeches and file them for reference.

As far as possible, guest speakers should come from the community itself. Parents should also be sought out as guest speakers. They should be given the latest material on the topic they will speak about so that they can do some research and thus present reasoned judgements.

Home Visits

Home visits are adequately covered dealt in the *Parents as Teachers Manual* compiled by LABCEC. It is available at LABCEC (for address see introduction). This manual was adapted from the Missouri's Parents as Teachers Programme for the ages of birth – three[6] and from Janet Browne's manual for the ages of 3-5.[7] J. Beaty also serves as an important reference.[8] The manual was funded by International Community Educators Association (ICEA). Although the manual has been adapted, it is based on the LABCEC experience.

From the initial home visits, it emerged that parents were clearly interested in learning how and what their children learnt at school. Thus it came about that instructional processes, considered important by the parents, were married to child development and growth, considered important by the centre, to make up the bulk of the programme. As noted, the programme and its activities are discussed in detail in the manual, which is obtainable in part or in whole from LABCEC at a cost of EC$.15 cents per photocopied page. A parent educator visiting a home of a 0-3 year old, for example, will follow these procedures:

A. Rapport Establishment
B. Observation
C. Discussion with parent
D. Lesson with parent and child
E. Summary.

At home, the parent educator will then write a report on the home visit which will include name of family, name and age of child, date of visit, topic, lesson, special problems and detailed, precise minutes of the home visit.[9]

Parent educators can be drawn from trained unemployed parents, social workers and early childhood education teachers. The most essential qualities of a Parent Educator are:

ability to communicate with people

experience with child-rearing processes

ability to establish rapport with the socio-economic group being visited.

Training of the parent educator should involve:

1. Orientation to the role of Parent Educator, including a discussion of the goals and objectives of the programme, an explanation of its justification, and a presentation of who will be visited and what will be the services provided. The manual should be read and explained in detail.

2. Training related to attitudes toward home visiting, including sensitivity to the needs and feelings of others and clarification of the parent educator's value system in relation to the socio-economic, ethnic and religious background and life styles of the people to be visited. Communication skills are extremely important, including the facilitation of communication among adults and children, communication with a headteacher or distraught parent and non-verbal communication.

3. Training related to skills and information needed on the job, including information on local groups that can be called on for assistance, knowledge of the materials to be taken on a home visit, the process of filling out forms, what to do and what not to do on a home visit, advice on acceptable manners in the home of a parent and rules of confidentiality about what is seen, heard and confided.

4. Detailed training on the PAT manual with particular reference to: 'What's special about this age?', 'What to look for?' in the different developmental areas, 'Things you can do to help' and the handouts for parents.

5. Before making a visit alone, the newly trained parent educator should accompany an experienced educator on a visit.

6. Continuous training is essential. At least once every two months, parent educators should liaise with the Director of the Centre and discuss written reports on their minutes and comments on the same. This discussion could be by telephone. Without this ongoing built-in training the programme will not last long.

Both parents and children value the Parents as Teachers programme highly. Parents report positive changes in attitudes, behaviours and actions. Parent educators report the same.

Up to now, some of the problems encountered during home visits have been serious. Parents have financial problems, live in minute homes, do not have enough food to feed their children adequately, need jobs, have problems with their relationships with their children's fathers, take drugs. In extreme cases, children are physically abused. There are other problems. Parents would like to have access to books and toys for their children. Parents shout at or beat children excessively.

Attempts should be made to provide solutions. Often, local or national groups can be contacted to give food-aid, clothes-aid or even financial help in certain instances. Local groups can be contacted to assist with adequate housing. Books and toys are being loaned to the parents. Additional counselling is needed for the parent and physically abused child. Parents are being counselled on the absolute necessity of at least one member of the household speaking to the child in English language all the time, although parents in Saint Lucia should be reminded that creole is their mother-tongue and, as such, should be valued and also spoken to the child. However, a referral system now being set into place needs to be systematised and formalised on the level of community to community.

Parents as Volunteers

Parents or other community members serving as volunteers should undergo training. They must be perfectly acquainted with the accreditation procedures and licensing requirements and these should be studied in depth. The curriculum and samples of activity sheets should also be accessible to and understood by the parents. In addition, these parents should read from cover to cover the *Parents as Teachers* manual. They should attend regular group meetings and membership meetings. They should also participate in training sessions relating to child development and growth on a yearly basis.

Parents also serve as volunteers – and very willingly – on field trips. They can also help in the creation of new learning materials and learning centres. Parents can tutor large and small groups, help on lunch duty and in extra-curricular activities. They can perform clerical activities such as grading and recording, filling out records and forms, as well as helping to maintain library books and learning files. Other community volunteers can also do these duties. Parents and other community volunteers can help to make the local and culturally relevant materials needed for each term.

In conjunction with the home visit programme, parents who have financial needs can be identified. Some cannot afford to send their children to the centre. Likewise, the centre has needs which the early childhood staff are hard-pressed to fill. Some of these needs are for assistants on playground duty. Very often, children do not get enough playground time, partly because they have other priorities and partly because the staff see playground duty as merely a supervisory task. Having a parent as a volunteer with a stipend to do daily playground duty for an hour or more per day is one way of ensuring that children's needs for outdoor play are met, that parents' needs for financial assistance and communication with their children are satisfied, and that staff needs for extra time can be catered for.

In addition, staff often find it difficult to come to the centre at the time the parents require. A parent or other community volunteer who comes in from 6.30am to

8.00am per day can do an indispensable service for the parents, staff and children. These small and financially strapped centres can also hardly afford the desirable ratios of staff to children. This is where a parent or two who come in for an hour or so to help bathe, dress, comb the children's hair and teach as parent volunteers can help immeasurably without driving up the costs of the operation too much. In fact, almost 100% of the volunteers are willing to function as full time volunteers. After three years of volunteerism, and with relevant training, full-time volunteers should be upgraded to teacher assistants.

Parent Teacher Conferences

Parent-teacher conferences or meetings are an important part of the school's programme. These can often be incorporated into open days. Projects should be displayed for viewing. Folders for each child should be ready, with examples of work done in the class. The Administrator and staff should prepare the specific topics they will talk about to each parent. They should greet the parent warmly and talk for a few minutes to get to know them and their hopes and dreams for their children. The Administrator and staff should take care not to begin the conference with negative remarks about the children. On the contrary, their first reaction should be to make positive comments and to let the parents, too, make positive comments. Any difficulties experienced by the child should be left for last and be discussed with great sensitivity for the parents' feelings about their child.

A conference should have a follow-up. Parents should be asked for a time for the next conference. One advantage of these conferences is that the parents can see that the Administrator and staff care about their child. There are clarifications to problems, issues. Advice is possible. Parents and children are encouraged to continue to do their best. Programmes can be extended and new plans formulated.

In all this, the treatment of the parents is extremely important. Parents must also see themselves as decision-makers, hence the suggestion that parents make up at least one-fourth of the board. Parents must feel welcome. They must feel that the staff, board and membership appreciate them. Parents must not feel that they are working at odds with the centre. Where there is an issue with which staff and parents do not agree, such as spanking or the writing of names, all efforts must be made to conciliate the parents and treat their opinions with respect. The staff should not be afraid of the parents. They should not be hostile to them or fearful of losing control. Nor should they feel that they are the trained professionals and the parents simply the 'botherers'. Staff should remember clearly that parents want the best for their children. Staff should conduct yearly parent evaluations in terms of parents' attitudes and their opinions of the centre. Where the account is negative, staff should not respond negatively but, rather, try to look at the errors made and see how these can be corrected.

Where parents and staff and board and membership all work in harmony and peace, this is one of the most important attributes of a quality centre is achieved.

Chapter 3

The role of the Director

The Director is the central figure in this non-governmental, not-for-profit institution. In many cases the Director's duties could be done by the Administrator. (In this case, 'Administrator' means the founding member and, most often, proprietor of the centre). Without the Director, the community emphasis of the work would be non-existent. If she or he does the work inadequately, the community's philosophy will be inadequate.

Care must be taken in choosing a Director from the local community. If the Director is not the initiator of the project, they should be chosen by the board, initiated either by the Early Childhood Education Administrator or by some advisor to the project. The Director would feel the pulse of the community on sensitive and important issues, know potential volunteers, help recruit potential staff and so on.

It is not important that Directors be Early Childhood Education professionals in these small Caribbean communities. However, they should be very well read on early childhood education and seek the advice of the Administrator whenever in doubt on any matter.

Directors should oversee board meetings. They should strive for a 60-70% turnout at board meetings. If the turnout is less, then either the Director is not relating to board members well enough, informing them early enough and reminding them of meetings, or members of the board have to be replaced. More often than not, once the board is committed, it is the Director who must provide leadership and who must review their tactics. It is essential that an agenda, along with accompanying papers including the past minutes, be circulated at least ten days in advance of the Board meeting. Board members need to come to the meetings prepared, so this is essential.

Topics which the Director should include on agendas of board meetings are:

- Classroom observation by parent field officers (every meeting)

- Constitution (at an initial meeting and for as many subsequent meetings as necessary)

- Licensing requirements (annually)

- Evaluation of Board members by each other, including their fund-raising performance and annual attendance.

- Board manual (annually)

- Letters to sponsors and follow-up (every meeting)

- Minutes of parent meetings (every meeting)

- Minutes of PAT (Parents as Teachers) home visits meetings (every meeting)

- Written policies of the centre (annually or as needed)

- Friends organisation (as needed)

- Job descriptions of Director and staff (annually)

- Annual budget (annually)

- Results of staff evaluations (annually)

- Annual report (annually)

- Discussions of parent questionnaires and follow-up.

- More casual annual evaluation of staff

- Forms of technical assistance to the Early Childhood Education Centres (ongoing).

For a more complete list of topics see the section on 'Agendas' on page 44.

At every meeting, the possible date or week of the next meeting should be set. The Director should then contact each Board member personally to confirm the date for the meeting. Agendas should then be sent ten days in advance and announcing the date of the meeting. A written reminder should be posted and a reminder by telephone should be made, whenever possible. Only if Directors follow the preceding steps with every board member, can they be absolved of the responsibility of low turnout. This excludes, of course, the Director's style at meetings, which should be democratic enough to encourage board attendance.

The Director, together with the Early Childhood Education Administrator, should be responsible for recruitment of staff for the centre. In cases where the Early

Childhood Education Administrator is not yet adequately trained, that is three years' training by relevant institutions, this duty should be done in conjunction with the Project Advisor where there is one. It is important that the board does not implicate itself in this recruitment. The board recruits the Director who, with the Early Childhood Education Administrator, recruits the staff. The board can advise or suggest staff members, but should not interfere with the actual recruitment or dismissal, although explanations for any dismissal should be given to the Board, and staff members should be given an opportunity to appeal to the Board.

Together with the Early Childhood Education Administrator, the Director should conduct yearly staff evaluations and the results should be presented to the Board. In addition, the Director should help the Early Childhood Education Administrator direct and hold parent meetings once a month. The Director should also coordinate parent volunteers. Parent volunteers such as the aide who arrives at 6.00a.m or 7a.m to facilitate parents who need to go to work early and works until the first member of staff comes in, or the volunteer who helps with the daycare or playground time should be used. These volunteers can ideally be poor parents who need the finance. The attendance of such parents at parent meetings should be compulsory for at least three consecutive years as part of their training. More importantly, these parents should be drawn from those who participated in the home visit programme for at least ten months, again to ensure a minimum level of training. In cases where the parent volunteers do not speak English, individual training should be given in Creole.

Another duty of the Director is to co-ordinate the Parents as Teachers home visit programme. The Director and the board should see PAT home visits as a priority since it has been proved that an early childhood education programme without community and parent involvement loses its value to the children.[10] Board members and membership should be encouraged to pay at least one home visit per month. The Director should hold bi-monthly meetings with the Parent Educators, where the contents of the home visits are discussed and the follow-up to problems instituted in the form of referral or other means.

Financial management oversight is also provided by the Director. There could be two separate account books – one for the Early Childhood Education Centre and one for fund-raising as coordinated by the Director. Ideally, however, one book is preferable. The Director should check the accounts on a monthly basis and produce monthly statements, ensuring that the line items are kept within the parameters of the annual budget. Also, along with the Early Childhood Education Administrator, the Director should ensure proper maintainance of the centre. Likewise, the Ministry's licensing requirements, a copy of which should be procured from the Ministry, should be met.

Preparing an annual report is essential. Without annual reports, much of the direction of the centre may be lost and the centre could fall foul of its objectives and activities. This annual report should include:

a. An explicit narrative description of the organisation's major activities including:

I. The early childhood education programme which should include:

- numbers registered for the year

- number of activity plans presented by each staff member every year. (They are expected to present these for the first three consecutive years of work only.

II. The parents' meetings, including:

- topics covered and guest speakers

- issues raised by parents

- follow-up.

III. The home visitation programme including:

- number of parents and children visited

- ages of children

- topics covered

- highlights of programme

- problems encountered with parents and children

- follow-up.

IV. Any other programme conducted by the centre.

V. A financial summary, describing:

Parents' fees
Fund-raising
Grants
Bank costs in
Loans in
Bank charges
Materials
Premises
Personnel

Food programme
Equipment
Miscellaneous

- A list of Board and staff members

- Audited financial statements or a comprehensive financial summary identifying revenues in the categories described above and reporting ending balances (when annual report does not include full audited financial statements, it should indicate that they are available on request).

The Director should assist the Project Advisor in liaising with funding agencies. The Director should sign all project proposals sent out and should be the signatory for all correspondence with all funding agencies – or the chairperson should be. Directors should, at minimum, read all project proposals and correspondence sent out. It is important that Directors be the signatories. It is helpful to the grantee organisation not to be associated with one agency or one Project Advisor making a request on behalf of a number of organisations. However, where it is strategically essential for the Project Advisor to sign a document, he or she should do so. Liaising with the Government is a highly important task of the Director. Government sets policy directions that to a large extent determine the activities of the centre; specific Ministries have a key role to play in areas of training and financial support, and their moral support is highly desirable. It can be counter-productive to the institution if such support is not given. Regular contact with relevant officials in the Ministries of Education, Planning, Health and Community Development in cases of needs only, can only assist the Director. All efforts should be made, if possible, to avoid conflict with officials of these Ministries.

Holding an Annual General Meeting, although a special event, does not need to involve much extra work for the Director. The AGM should involve a meeting of Board, staff, parents, general membership or friends of the centre, sponsors and desirable outside persons. For the AGM, an advance agenda with written reports should be provided. There should be a time schedule which should be adhered to. Time should be left for questions, discussions and debate. The AGM should be topped up with a fun-filled and interesting activity. The Director and Board should remember that the chosen speaker should fit into the mainstream of their current efforts. Plans should be carefully laid to honour and recognise those who have served faithfully. Where possible, interesting locations should be selected for AGMs and the Director and Board should work hard at promoting attendance. A fee should be charged for lunch or dinner. A telephone campaign should be conducted to promote attendance. Advance notices should be sent to the media. A committee should be appointed from the Board. The tasks – registration, promotion, awards, programme, publicity – should be distributed. Finally, special attention should be paid to the arrangements of the AGM.[11]

One of the major roles of the Director is to oversee the membership or friends of the centre. The members of the centre comprise friends of staff, board or parents who are associated with the centre in some way or the other. Along with the Administrator, the Director should hold staff meetings at least once every two months, of which records should be kept. The Director is also responsible for the preparation of annual budgets and for ensuring a yearly audit.

In fact, Directors need to be responsible for a number of centres and operate as Community Cluster Organisers. The duties of the Director could then be divided up between the Director or Community Cluster Organiser and the various Administrators. To repeat, for emphasis: many of the Director's duties could be done by an Administrator.

Where no Director can initially be found, duties could be divided up among two or three board members. This should, however, be seen as temporary because a dedicated and committed leader is one of the signs of a successful not-for-profit organisation.

The Director's role can be an exciting and stimulating one. It is a dedicated role. However, the staff, Board and membership should remember clearly that the Director's role is, in part, a volunteer one – one which requires hard work and a great deal of commitment. The Director must be supported and not treated cynically. It should be appreciated clearly by all involved that inextricably embedded in the Director's duties is loads of community love.

Chapter 4

The role of other stakeholders

The early childhood education administrator

Like the Director, the Early Childhood Education Administrator's role is crucial – but for different reasons. As noted in the previous section, the Director and the Administrator could be one and the same. The Administrator also determines the community ethos, particularly through interaction with the parents. Parent interaction, discussed in a previous section, applies also to the Administrator. The Administrator is vital in determining, more than anyone else, the spirit of the centre.

Administrators should be trained. This is crucial to their conducting proper work. They should have undergone at least three years training at relevant institutions. If this training is not complete, they should be in the process of completion. Under no circumstances should there be an Administrator who is neither trained nor applying to be properly trained.

One of the duties of Early Childhood Education Administrators is to organise and supervise work, through writing and supervising the daily activity plans. This is important as it forms part of the staff training. They should also do supervised activities with a group of children, i.e. 'teach' for about two hours per day, keeping records of the children's work as they do so. The Administrator is, along with the Director, responsible for maintaining the centre and for animating annual events such as Christmas parties, Graduations, Open Days and so on. Attendance records, meeting the Ministry's licensing requirements, and sitting on the Board are all part of the Administrator's duties. The Administrator should set aside two hours per week for training other staff members. This training could include:

–   The *Parents as Teachers* manual

–   Licensing requirements

–   Classroom observation

–   Topics from the curriculum

–   Excerpts from this Handbook

–   Self study

–   Preparation of a newsletter

–   First aid

–   Forms of technical assistance

–   National Insurance Scheme

–   Involvement of fathers

–   Writing activity plans

–   Other topics on child development.

Early Childhood Education Administrators should help Directors liaise with the Ministries. Importantly, they should collect, or supervise the collection of, all fees as well as entering all receipts and payments in the accounting book. In some centres, this responsibility could be delegated to another staff member, an office assistant, for example. When this is done, however, Administrators should peruse the books at least once per term. They should acquaint themselves with the monthly statements and, where amounts are higher than proposed in the annual budgets, take all steps to make these amounts balance with the budget. Administrators should do or supervise postage, payment of NIS, transactions with the bank; they should make sure that all bills such as electricity, telephone, water and rent are paid promptly.

However, perhaps the crux of Early Childhood Education Administrators' duties is their interaction with the children. Since they do not do this alone but as part of the responsibilities shared by all staff members, this topic is dealt with in the next section.

The Administrator has authority over the rest of the staff but must take care that this is not abused. Harsh administration will almost inevitably be counter-productive. If authority is excersised with firmness yet gentleness, it will slowly become clear to the other members of staff that the Administrator is in control and the staff members will respond, according the respect that is deserved.

The term 'in control' must itself be used with caution. Administrators really should be in control of themselves and in control when situations are difficult but not necessarily in control of others. Others are not to be controlled or manipulated. Rather, they are to be understood. Administrators have to treat every member of staff as an equal – deserving of respect. In this way, respect will be returned.

This does not mean that Administrators do not have the right and duty to exert their authority when decisions have to be made. The decisions may be painful to some but necessary to ensure the discipline of the institution. The decisions should be taken firmly but gently, and in no case should Administrators try to take revenge on a member of staff or to exert authority with undue harshness. This attitude will be resented by others and they will react in ways inimical to the interest of the institution and to the Early Childhood Education Administrator.

One problem which resurfaces is the matter of sharing the day to day tasks such as cleaning. In certain cases, Administrators complain that staff are not pulling their weight. In others, staff complain that Administrators are not pulling theirs. Administrators must strike a balance. Early Childhood Education Administrators, like other staff members, are supposed to help in the cleaning up. The staff are only servants to the extent that Administrators themselves are servants. In cases where the staff is not helping enough, Administrators must demand firmly that they do so. However, it might be useful for Administrators also to examine their own practice. Do they lead by example? Do they pull their weight in helping? What are their relations with staff? Are they so good that the staff feel like cooperating? Are staff relations handled in a balanced manner? Or is administration sometimes too harsh and sometimes too soft and lax, causing confusion in the minds of the staff members, leading to disrespect when administrators are too 'soft' and resentment when an administrator suddenly tries to make up for 'softness' by being too harsh. Posted schedules, firmly and gently implemented, can help deal with this problem.

The conduct of good relations with one's staff is not an easy task. Personalities clash even if there are no other problems. In cases where characters clash or there is an open quarrel around a work issue, great sensitivity and care are needed. While insisting on the work that needs to be done, no anger should be shown, nor hasty and negative things said about the other, even if the staff member's anger gets out of hand and bitter things are said. In fact, it might be a good opportunity for the Administrator later, in private, to question whether criticisms expressed in anger by staff members were unjust or just.

When unjust criticisms are made by staff members to Administrators, a face-to-face session in private, when emotions have calmed down – and certainly not on the same day – is needed to sort matters out. On the other hand, if the Administrator is at fault, they should most certainly apologise.

As noted before, the conduct of good relations between the Administrators and staff is not easy. To succeed, Administrators must treat staff as persons deserving of respect, and be understanding, kind and patient. They must be responsive to the moods of the staff and try their best to cooperate with the staff – but not if this means not upholding the levels of quality that the institution requires. In other words, Administrators should not give in to the staff when this can be to the detriment of the institution, including the children.

In their relations, the Early Childhood Education Administrators determine the tone of the centre in relation to parents, staff and children. It is a unique role, one of great responsibility. In this, every Administrator must be a role model.

The role of the other staff

Staff is extremely important. Parents are extremely concerned with the quality of care their children receive at a centre, and it is the staff who determine this quality. A staff member who speaks harshly or shouts at the children, is rough with the parents, chats often with friends outside the centre or sends children's clothes home with faeces on them, is working to the detriment of the institution. On the other hand, a trained staff member who demonstrates great qualities of kindness, love, patience, caring, stability and joy in their work is an asset to the institution.

The staff should draw up daily activity plans for as long as it takes them to master this activity. Even when staff members have completed a full set of perfect plans based on the curriculum, they should still do an agreed minimum of new, creative plans per month. Records should be kept of children's work to send home. The staff should attend and help to animate all parents' meetings. They should attend regular training sessions, organised by the centre, the Ministries and other personal development and academic training institutes. Where, for instance, continuing education in CXC English and Math are available, staff might enrol. Shopping – as delegated by the Administrator – paying NIS, doing bank trans-actions and paying electricity, telephone and water bills promptly are all part of staff responsibilities. In some instances, staff may have to receive parental fees. Keeping the premises clean (kitchen, bathroom, mirrors, sinks, yards, bedsheets) and recording food items used are staff duties. Each member of staff, including the Administrator, should pay at least one home visit per year to parents, dividing the registered parents among the staff on roll.

Interaction among staff and children is tremendously important. Staff should interact frequently with the children, demonstrating their affection, interest and respect.[12] They should interact not only orally but also by smiling, touching and holding. They should talk with and listen to children individually during activities and routines. They should seek meaningful conversations with them. Staff should give one-to-one attention to infants during feeding and diapering, allowing time for the infants to respond. Staff should be available and responsive to the children. They should quickly comfort infants in distress, reassure crying toddlers, listen to children with attention and respect, and respond to their questions and requests. Staff should be aware of the activities of the entire group even when dealing with a smaller group. They should position themselves strategically and look up often from whatever they are doing. They should spend time observing each child without interrupting an actively involved child.

The staff should speak with children in a friendly, courteous manner. They should speak with individual children often and should include children in conversations. They should speak to children at eye level and call children by name. The staff should encourage children of all ages to use language. They should treat children of all races, religions, family backgrounds and cultures with equal respect and consideration. They should provide girls and boys with equal opportunities to take part in all activities. For example, they should provide models, props and visual images that counter traditional sex-role limitations, such as female firefighters and male nurses. Staff should value positive levels of noise and activity involving both girls and boys. When acknowledging individual children, staff should avoid gender stereotypes in language references. They should use words such as strong, gentle, beautiful, helpful for both boys and girls. Grouping children by gender should be avioded.

The independence of children as they become ready should be encouraged by the staff. Staff should use positive approaches to help children behave constructively. Guidance methods should include redirecting, planning ahead to prevent problems, encouraging appropriate behaviour and developing consistent, clear rules in conjunction with children, discussed with them to make sure they understand, and then consistently enforced. Staff should describe the situation to encourage children's evaluation of any problem rather than impose a solution. They should never use physical punishment or other negative discipline methods that hurt, frighten or humiliate children.

Children should be generally comfortable, relaxed, happy and involved in play and other activities. Children should not be silent but should sound happy and purposeful. The staff should help children deal with anger, sadness and frustration by comforting, identifying and reflecting upon their feelings and helping the children use words to solve their problems. They should encourage children in social behaviours such as cooperating, helping, taking turns and talking to solve problems. It is important that the staff model the desired behaviours among themselves. Staff expectations of children's social behaviour should be developmentally appropriate. For example, infants should interact freely with one another while the staff observe them, alert to respond and model safe interaction when necessary. Pre-schoolers should be encouraged to cooperate in small groups. Children should be encouraged to talk about feelings and ideas instead of trying to resolve problems with force.

A quality centre means a caring centre. A caring centre automatically demands a caring staff. Staff must be trained in appropriate behaviours and appropriate attitudes for a quality environment at the centre to be sustained.

Technical Assistance

Technical assistance is only essential when an Early Childhood Education Administrator would like to start a community-run centre but does not yet have a functioning Director or Board. However, it is important to note that technical assistance is also essential in instances where an Early Childhood Education Centre needs financial backup from funding agencies in order to achieve a level of quality in terms of areas such as building, resource materials and training. Technical assistance may be needed to train the Director, Administrator, staff, parents and other community members.

Tapping into international sources of funding is another reason for technical assistance. Assistance does not have to come from the Director's local community. It will be needed by the institution only until the institution is financially and intellectually self-sustainable, a feat which may take between two and seven years to accomplish.

Technical assistance could be sought from an institution or from someone who holds, at minimum, a BA degree. He or she should communicate easily with others and, especially, be able to tap into foreign sources of funding. Nevertheless, this assistance should not be seen only as a lead into foreign funding sources. The person or institution chosen should be able to provide the technical assistance to foster successful growth in the quality of the organisation. In other words, this technical assistance should assist the Director in terms of setting up a quality institution. The institution or chosen person serves as an important additional trained human resource who can aid the Director – for a period of time – in establishing a quality Early Childhood Education Centre.

It is likely to entail acquiring land and building, since suitable low-cost accommodation is rare in this island. The institution or person providing this technical assistance will need access to a computer and require skills at letter-writing and preparing proposals.

Technical assistance can also be useful to the Director in:
- construction
- training
- financial management assistance
- Parents as Teachers Programme with home visits
- other parental involvement activities
- setting up a local board of management
- research and purchasing play equipment and resource accoutrements
- networking
- field visits
- membership
- other.

The indispensability of such technical assistance lies in the institution's or person's access to foreign funding agencies and their ability to pass on experience gained from establishing or working with one community-run institution, to the members and officers of other institutions. It is a necessity which has a time-span – because a local community-run institution which remains dependent on a central institution for its management is not really managed by the community and does not impart real ownership to the community. Good technical assistance initiates successful projects in communities, projects which are surviving without the institution or person. In other words, a good technical assistant or project advisor is just passing by and leaves in their wake successful community-managed and owned, sustainable institutions.

The Board

There are manifest benefits in having a board, including the enormous advantage of contributing to financial sustainability. Finance should, however, not be the only or major reason for having a board. No board member would accept the enormous fund-raising responsibilities without a strong moral, intellectual, social, emotional and creative commitment to the institution. Getting such great commitment, and attracting board members away from other volunteer activities, requires a great deal of hard work, dedication, time and commitment on the part of the Director and the Pre-School Administrator.

Board members should be people who are admired, respected and inspiring. They need not be chosen by only one person, although this is inevitable when there is only one founding member. Ideally, however, where there are two or three founding members, they can form a nominating committee for board members. Where the board is already functioning, the board itself should form a nominating committee to choose incoming board members. Where even the nominating committee is uncertain about whom to choose, it is advisable to seek the advice of religious and community group leaders. In recruiting a new board member, one should send an attractive letter, carried and presented, if possible, by an impressive delegation. Even if the invitation is turned down, some important public relations work would have been achieved.

Board members should be people with special human qualities of kindness, patience, love, community spirit, dedication, commitment and intelligence. They should have the respect of the community, and unpopular people should be avoided. This does not mean that the board members chosen will not have enemies but they should have such strength of character that the balance of popularity weighs clearly on their side. Some board members with enormous human spirit may not necessarily be popular in the sense that the politician is popular, for example. However, they should at least hold the respect of the local community and, in the case of an employer, have the reputation for fairness and integrity.

Human qualities, although enormously important, are not the only basis for choosing a board member. There is at least one Caribbean organisation which is extremely developed, sophisticated and genuinely caring, that adopts the policy that board members should come from the non-influential sections of the local community. O'Connell confirms this policy by stating that if one wants to change the *status quo* it is inadvisable to choose members from the *status quo*.[13] On national and governmental level this attitude has sound reason behind it, but on the local community level it might be wise to apply alternative criteria.

On the local community level, in the field of early childhood education, indispensable potential allies are, for example, the principal of the local Infant or Primary Schools. So is the District Education Officer of the area. A principal or district education officer nominated by the Ministry does not reach this position without personal qualities of leadership, determination and flexibility. Nevertheless, the fact remains that these individuals may be required to alter their philosophies slightly.

Leaders of youth organisations are also important allies. Some youth may well feel uncomfortable working with older people. However, persistence should be maintained so that youth leaders are adequately represented on the board. In the case of Saint Lucia, the same applies to minorities in terms of race, religion or nationality. Former Government officials with the human qualities described above, presently working in the private or public sector can be a source of enormous strength. Business should be allied as well. Business people can offer remarkable acumen and they demand the kind of accountability and efficiency which is not the forte of two-thirds of the not-for-profit organisations, according to O'Connell – who asserts that one-third of not-for-profit organisations are average in their efficiency and one-third poor.[14] The object is to appoint influential people who are committed, dedicated and enthusiastic, and who bring about changes in attitudes in a community with a rapidity that non-influential people cannot achieve.

However, so-called 'non-influential' people, common folk and the poor, must have a place, and they do. Sometimes, particularly in rural communities, people of a lesser socio-economic level including teachers and nurses may make up the bulk of the Board – but they might well constitute the elite of that rural community. Parents should be automatically elected by other parents to the Board and should make up at least one-fourth of the board. The parents elected might not come from the dispossessed of the society. The board must always have some dispossessed people or those from the lowest socio-economic strata. These people have a unique experience which they can share. They often incorporate extreme views mirroring the community views, both negative and positive – so positive that sometimes they serve as the soul of the board. It is important that they are not so sparsely respresented on the board that they become the silent minority.

There are times when Board members will not agree. At times like this, it is quite useless to remark that although they have different opinions they really have a common approach. The chair should certainly note the disagreement. Equally important, the matter should be brought to the vote. Board members should not hesitate to vote over issues which are important. A matter which is important and controversial enough should be discussed in at least two board meetings before a decision is taken. It is better to lose, even on critical issues, as long as the organisation comes out of the fight with greater confidence in the integrity of the process.

A Board manual is essential. This should include the history of the organisation, by-laws, policies and important procedures, organisation charts, Board list, committee lists, a staff organisation chart with a summary of functions, current annual report, major programme activities and the home telephone numbers of Director, Early Childhood Education Administrator and Project Advisor.

The Board should not be afraid of turnover. If a board member, after one annual evaluation, is not contributing, the Chair of the Board should not hesitate to write a letter pointing out that a majority of responsibilities have not been met – which should be listed – and noting that if the person is too busy otherwise, they should resign from board membership and join the ordinary membership i.e. the Friends of the institution. A Chairperson or Director who fails to do this will soon find that they have a non-functioning organisation which will become meaningless. In the responsibilities assigned to the Board member, it is worthwhile to insist upon the fund-raising aspect, although, as noted, this is only one area of a large commitment. Board members who do not help to raise funds must be replaced unless their commitment in the majority of other functions is so outstanding as to render their resignation inapproptiate. Only one or two such exceptions in each board can be made or it will not be possible for a quality early childhood institution to survive.

At the same time, it is important to reward good Board members. The Director or Administrator should not hesitate to call Board members regularly to say thank you. Plaques and pins should be distributed to committed board members at the Annual General Meeting or other such fora.

It may seem particularly difficult to mobilise and activate a Board. However, the Director or Early Childhood Education Administrator should not be discouraged. It is possible. It has been done before and the rewards are well worth the pain.

Financial sustainability and membership
It may seem strange to discuss financial sustainability in conjunction with membership but in a successfully run Early Childhood Education Centre the marriage is obvious. Most Early Childhood Education Administrators know the

financial difficulties related to their centres. For a few months of the year, especially July and August, many Administrators earn nothing. Unless a school is a high-income, profit oriented centre, Administration is often strapped for cash.

This is not a criticism of high-cost for-profit centres. They have their role in the society. However, the socio-economic status of the majority of the population means that this is not the path that most Early Childhood Education Centres can take. In terms of finance, there are three types of centres: the high-cost for-profit; the low-cost for-profit; and the low-cost or, better described: cost-effective not-for-profit.

The difference between the high-cost and the low-cost is evident. However, the difference between the two low-cost types: the for-profit and the not-for-profit is not so clear but it can be identified. The not-for-profit is run by a board of management whereas the for-profit is run by an individual. Also, the margin of profit in the not-for-profit is automatically fed back into the centres in the form of materials, resource accoutrements and so on whereas the margin of profit in the for-profit, in the case of the low-cost centre, that is fed back into these items depends entirely on the individual owner. Again, this is certainly not an attempt to discredit any type of centre. Nevertheless, it should be noted that between the cost-effective not-for-profit and the low-cost for-profit, quality is lkely to be on the side of the not-for-profit. A successful cost-effective not-for-profit, community-run centre should be a goal of the low-cost schools, if, that is, the centre is community-run.

Typically, the majority of income for these centres comes from the parents' fees – between 80 and 90%. Government should recognise its commitment to early childhood education including the continuing education component of parenting education, within the limitations of government, and give some financial help to each of the low-cost, not-for-profit, community-run centres. However, Government will only pay attention after a broad base has been built up. So, if a small organisation finds itself knocking against a wall in terms of getting financial support from government, instead of trying to force the wall – which will only result in damage to the small non-governmental institution, it is probably wiser to withdraw even if only for a while, concentrate on fund-raising through membership and work on becoming a part of a vibrant, broad-based organisation which will be able to influence government much more.

For financial sustainability in the cost-effective not-for-profit organisations in developing Caribbean countries where governments do not or cannot give fully adequate financial support to early childhood education centres, the role of the membership in fund-raising is crucial. Fund-raising is important even for the other types of institutions but fund-raising through membership is rendered difficult if not impossible for them by the fact that they are not community-run.

This is not to deny the other forms of fund-raising – cake sales, dances, raffles and so on – however, in many of these cases, much effort is expended for little financial gain. The role of the membership is an important way of altering the balance in favour of the institution.

Membership organisations do not necessarily flourish successfully in the Caribbean. Important exceptions are the Mothers and Fathers Associations in Saint Lucia and this offers positive hope for membership organisations. There is a catch to making a membership organisation flourish. If members are selected at random and asked to join an organisation, the organisation might well fail. The members should have some common focus initially, until their commitment to early childhood education gradually develops. It is suggested that this common focus be a person whom they admire – a best or good friend or a close relative. Accordingly the board, parents and staff should be asked to name a few of of their best friends or relatives from the community. These friends or relatives should be asked by the board to join the organisation, sent a letter signed by this same member with whom they are associated, explaining the reasons why they are being asked to join the organisation, and they should, thirdly, be reminded by this same Board member of the meeting date. It is important to realise from the outset that this will be a long, painstaking task. However, the effort expended on it will not be greater than the effort expended on other fund-raising and the results in terms of fund-raising, community participation, community education and relations, government advocacy and so on, will be far more.

It is vital to realise that one distinct function of the membership will be to fund-raise. Members will raise funds partly or even principally by finding donors who will donate to the institution on an annual basis. In Saint Lucia, it has been proven that a board can successfully raise funds of EC$10,000.00 a year this way. However, for the membership to fund-raise, there must be an element of seriousness involved. The Board must not be afraid to turn over its membership gently. If a member has not even raised even one donor for one year, they should be sent a letter about this and reprimanded by their board friend. If for two years running, members have still not produced even one donor, they should be asked to resign and may well be happy to do so and be replaced. It is important to do this. Of course if the member is contributing greatly in other spheres, this rule may be waived. However, it should be waived in consultation with the rest of the board and in very few cases or else the organisation might well collapse.

It is the purpose and importance of the organisations mission that will give the purpose and thrust to the membership. The goal – in this case the crucial importance of early childhood education – must be seriously worked on. Each membership meeting should be an opportunity to educate the members on the vital importance of early childhood education to human development and therefore the vital importance of their contribution to early childhood education. Meetings will be enhanced by good guest speakers. They should, as much as possible, come from the community and be well informed on the topic they present.

The membership should be clearly aware of its functions. These functions include:

Clarifying the institution's mission

Sensitising the community on early childhood education including parenting

Enhancing the public image

Advocating the interests of the centre with government

Approving long-range plans

Assessing the performance of the membership

Ensuring financial solvency

Each function will need careful elaboration on how it will be approached.

Finally, in the mobilisation of the membership, the Director and the Early Childhood Education Administrator have a key role to play. The Director should have a high degree of personal development. Awareness of self and highly developed awareness of others is an asset. It should be evident to the membership or the volunteers that the Director is making sacrifices – going well beyond the call of duty. Members may even express some feelings of guilt in terms of the level of commitment of the Director but this guilt should not be encouraged as it may turn to resentment. Rather, it should be channelled in positive directions.

It is important that Directors have precise a understanding of people and of themselves. They should not assume that they are appreciated all of the time. The Director may be loved sometimes but certainly not all of the time. Human relations are much more complex. It is extremely important that Directors give the membership praise and reinforce members' self-esteem. They should draw the membership closer by calling volunteers by name often. Directors should let each volunteer know that they are valued and praise all efforts made. Volunteers should feel needed, useful and that their Director feels that they are important in the eyes of the Director and all the membership.

On the other hand, no Director should push this positive reinforcement to the extreme of a lie. It is important to let volunteers know gently when they are failing in their functions as community volunteers. It is important that this is done gently and only once a year during the assessment, or volunteers might regretfully withdraw. This cannot be stressed too much. Volunteers cannot be beaten into participation. However, Directors should not pander to the negative vibrations received from any volunteer and should at all costs learn to recognise evil intentions and avoid them.

Eye contact is very important. A community volunteer may be making a point far removed from any personal comment on the Director but may look in the Director's eyes while mentioning a certain word. This may seem irrelevant but this volunteer is talking to the Director and not to someone else. The interaction between the Director and the volunteer is what matters most at that particular point, the volunteer constantly conveying messages about how they feel about the Director and what is being said at the moment. The Director should try to learn to understand the subtle messages being conveyed through eye contact and respond to them, so averting unnecessary blow-ups.

The use of interjection is also important. Knowing when to interject on particular words to convey suggestions, understanding the use of interjections by volunteers to convey criticism or self-criticism, is an art. As volunteers talk to their Director, they will be constantly agreeing or disagreeing with what the Director says and their interjections should be attended to with care.

Directors should be on the constant lookout for evidence of racism and xenophobia (fear of foreigners). Racial slurs may not be open but subtly present. Certainly, the best thing to do when they are not open is to ignore them. Subtlety, after all, is an expression of democracy. However, one way of countering such racism or xenophobia is to ensure that community membership reflect all racial, national and religious groups prevalent in the society. The Director should be a role-model in this humanising process.

Importantly, every Director must know when to keep quiet. If they have influenced a decision to advantage, they should not hammer home the contribution given. Keeping quiet or ignoring is also another way to respond to negative suggestions and hints from volunteers. Open disagreement on little matters is better avoided. Directors should save their energies for the big issues and handle smaller matters through action of the sort suggested above.

It is worth repeating that youth should be integrated into community movements. The Director and older community volunteers must recognise that they are mortal. They depend on the youth to continue their work and to create their own solutions. This work can only be continued and these problem-solving strategies conducted if this is understood and appreciated and if opportunities for creativity are presented to the youth. So the youth should be integrated as a vital part of the groups, and given responsibilities.

A love for oneself and for others is an invaluable aspect of all community work. Momentary self-hatred when we have committed an error and hatred of others when they have wounded us is part of the natural process of life. However, this should only be momentary. When a Director wounds involuntarily – they should not wound voluntarily, although this does not deny that criticism of others will be necessary at times – it is important that they make up for it by giving special recognition to the person concerned.

Community work is fragile. It is all about feelings and their management. People can feel hurt, upset, jealous or fearful. The best of people are sometimes devious, have evil intentions, are too 'soft' or too 'hard', are disrespectful, unruly, 'warrish'. These feelings must be managed by the Director and Administrator and brought onto a positive level. If not, community action will not survive. Repressive volunteer action simply does not exist.

Notes and References

1.   Alice S. Honig, *Parent Involvement in Early Childhood Education* (Washington, NAEYC, 1979) p. 8

2.   George S. Morrison, *Parent Involvement in the home, School and Community* (Columbus Toronto London Sydney, Charles E. Merrill Publishing Co., 1978) p. 7

3.   *Ibid*

4.   Heither B. Weiss, *Going to Scale: Issues in the Development and Proliferation of Community-Based Family Support and Education Programmes* (Cambridge, Massachusetts, Harvard Family Research Project, prepared for the Bernard Van Leer   Foundation, 1988)

5.   Morrison, *op. cit.* p. 127

6.   PAT Manual (Laborie, St. Lucia, LABCEC, 1993)

7.   Janet Brown, *The experience of Parenting* (Jamaica, Regional Pre-School Child Development Centre, Department of Extra-Mural Studies, U.W.I., 1984)

8.   Janice J. Beaty, *Observing Development of the Young Child.* second edition (New York, Merrill, 1990)

9.   Morrison, *op.cit.* p.127

10.   Alice S. Honig, *op. cit.* p. 8

11.   Brian O'Connel, *The Board Member's Book*, second edition (U.S.A., The Foundation Centre, 1985) pp. 101-104

12.   National Association for the Education of Young Children (NAEYC), *Guide to Accreditation* (Washington, NAEYC, 1991)

13.   O'Connel, *op.cit.*, p. 39

14.   *Ibid*, p. 163

Chapter 5

Agendas for board meetings of Caribbean community based Early Childhood Education Centres

Introduction

Board Agendas are important. Without them, there is an absence of planning. Without them, board members risk becoming bored at the repetitiveness of the agenda. The community board may become extinct.

In this document, it is assumed that community boards meet no more than once a month or once every two months.

This document is not meant to be read or used in isolation. It should be read along with the other sections of this handbook.

The following list of agendas and the detailed papers attached are by no means exhaustive. Board members may suggest many more topics for the agenda. This list was compiled over twelve years of working with community boards. It is hoped that it empowers community board members to conduct effective board meetings.

Agenda

1. Minutes

The first item on any agenda is the reading of the minutes. A secretary should be elected at the very first meeting. This secretary should be highly literate and should understand the importance the group attaches to her (or his) task. An assistant secretary should also be elected, who can act for the secretary if she is absent from a board meeting. Likewise the assistant should give the minutes to a board member if he or she will be absent.

The importance of the minutes cannot be stressed enough. Without these minutes there can be no follow-up of matters agreed upon by the board.

2. Errors and Omissions
No comments

3. Matters arising
No comments

4. Board Education
Board education should be done at every meeting on matters relating to early childhood education. LABCEC has materials for board education already prepared, and these can be consulted.

5. Board Policies
Board policies are the soul of Agendas. Board policies can be formulated on any and more of the policies below:

- **Finance**
  - Board budget policy
  - policy on compensation
  - policy on asset protection
  - policy on funding priorities
  - policy on building rental

- **Personnel**
  - policy on treatment of personnel
  - policy on compensation
  - policy on absences from work
  - policy on volunteers
  - policy on executive limitations
  - policy on budgeting

- **Ethics**
  - policy concerning prudence and ethics
  - policy on moral ownership

- **Administration**
  - policy on administrative clarity
  - policy on secretariats
  - policy on hurricanes and storms

- **Board**
  - policy on board meetings
  - policy on absent board members

- **Culture**
  - policy on Creole (where applicable)

Following is an example of one board's policy:

Board policy on parents who owe fees

The board recognises that many parents in Laborie cannot afford to pay the full cost for quality pre-school and daycare education. However, those who can afford to give donations in kind – such as farmers, fishermen and dressmakers – should do so. Those who cannot afford to give a donation in kind should give a donation in time such as serving as pre-school volunteers.

1. A parent should not owe LABCEC for more than one term

2. Any parent owing LABCEC for more than a term must either pay a visit to the Coordinator or write a letter to her

3. A parent who has not paid for three months must give payments in kind or time

4. All outstanding fees to LABCEC must be paid before graduation.

---

6. Follow up

The board and Administrator should list all items which need to be followed up by the Administrator and staff.

7. AOB

Any other business

8. Parent Educator minutes

Comments on Parent Educator minutes should be read at board meeting on boards where there is an active home visitation programme. These minutes are based on a manual available from LABCEC. The comments should be compiled by the Administrator or the Project Advisor. For an example of comments on minutes see Appendix 2 on page 59.

9. Friends and AGMs (Annual General Meetings)

Each board member should be asked to submit a list of names of their friends in the community, along with addresses and telephone numbers. The best strategy for collecting these names is to ask the board members to write them down during the meeting. These names should be given to the secretariat to be entered on computer and in filing boxes.

The functions of the friends are:

- Clarifying the mission of the institution or institutions

- Participating in an educational process on Early Childhood Education

- Enhancing the public image

- Advocating with government

- Approving long-range plans

- Assessing friends' performance

The friends together with the parents, sponsors and board members of the centres involved will make up the membership body. They should meet once per year for an AGM. Meetings more than once per year would cause difficulties of organisation for the secretariat and extra expense. These AGMs should discuss:

1. Annual budget of past and future year

2. Reports from the board

3. Elections of at least three friends to the board

4. Education on Early Childhood Education by qualified guest speaker

5. Education on other programmes of centres by qualified quest speaker

6. General discussion of friends

7. Cultural entertainment by children, parents and groups

8. AOB

9. Refreshments

The centres should contribute towards the cost for refreshments.

10. Absent board members

Some board members may persistently be absent without excuse. A board with less than 80% turnout is not an effective community board. Absent board members should not be alienated even after being absent for three consecutive meetings without an excuse, but should be supplemented although *not* replaced. That is, the board members should suggest another community member who will come to meetings regularly, while still continuing to write to the absent board member informing him or her of meetings. This is because the absent board member may, in fact, be a committed community volunteer at heart or at least, a possible friend.

After a board member has missed more than two meetings out of six without an excuse or three meetings out of 12, the board should consider replacing him or her permanently.

This supplementing and replacing of board members should be done assiduously if the board is to remain effective.

11. Board turnover

On any board there should be some turnover each year. This turnover could be no more than three members per year for continuity and these could be parents or friends. The fixed members of the board have, in LABCEC's case, served between 9 and 12 years without their commitment and contribution diminished. Fixed board members are essential in the Caribbean, where the scarcity of human resources is a problem. Each board should decide whether some members are in fact life-long members for as long as they hold their official positions such as Education Officer, for example, or Principals of Infant or Combined schools.

12. Scholarships

The plight of the poor in the community should be a matter of concern to the board. This is evident through the Parents as Teachers programme, where as many as 120 parents are visited per month, many of them poor. Also, many children aged from birth to five do not attend pre-schools/daycares. Boards should seek development of government policies concerning these mostly underprivileged children. Should Government, as Nimicht suggests,[1] create daycares where children attend twice per week and parents attend weekly sessions? There could be collaboration with already existing centres, whether private or government.

The boards could help to small extent through the provision of scholarships. Each centre should provide a minimum of scholarships per year and the board and secretariat should be encouraged to find sponsors for these underprivileged children.

13. Elections

The Chairperson and Secretary of the board should be influential people capable of negotiation with funders, government, business and private citizens. So there may not be a need to rotate the chairperson or secretary since such persons are in short supply, unless the need is felt. The treasurer likewise is very important, especially for accountability of overseas and local monies.

14. Brainstorming for proposals out (needs of centre)

Once a year, boards should brainstorm on proposals which the centre could try to write or could seek technical assistance from the national association to write. These proposals could concern building maintenance, toilets, conference facilities, building a resource room, playground equipment etc.

15. Reports on annual staff evaluations

Reports on annual staff evaluations of Administrator and board should be made at a full board meeting with staff and project advisor present, at least once per year. These evaluations should be based on the job description which should comprise initiative, perseverance, follow-up and community commitment as well as on sections of the self-study. See Appendix 7 for a sample questionnaire.

16. Reports on annual evaluations of children

These evaluations should be drawn up by the administrator, once per year and the results presented to the board.

17. Reports on self-study

A self-study of the centre should be done and the report presented to the board. See Appendices 7 and 8 for the primary material needed in the preparation of a narrative self-study.

18. Annual reports

Annual reports should be prepared by the secretariat along with the board members. They should be circulated to all board members and at least to sponsors.

19. Auditor's report

An auditor's report should be prepared once a year.

20. Report on policy monitoring

Each year at least three of the board's policies should be monitored to ensure that policies are being implemented. This monitoring can be done by the Administrator, the board or by an external evaluator. The monitoring should be strictly based on board policy.

21. Parents on board

The board should elect at least three parents on a 12 person board. At least one of these parents should be an underprivileged person. The board is not a parent board but a community one. The board should have at least one or two underprivileged persons on it for the full development of its compassionate nature and these members should be listened to and their views valued.

22. Report on common entrance results

The centre should follow up the common entrance results of the children who registered at the centre and, if possible, compare it with the averages in the community or with children who attended other pre-schools. For instance, LABCEC's common entrance for the first five years the children sat common entrance has been 81% minimum and 100% maximum.

23. Parents as Teachers programme

The board should read the short booklets on the PAT programme available at LABCEC. This will inform them about the justification, objectives and activities of the programme as well as about the concerns raised by parents and children.

24. Relations with other Pre-Schools/Daycares in the area

Pre-Schools/Daycares who are not involved in the community board should be constantly wooed for their involvement. They should be invited to all the board's functions including training sessions

25. Mission statement

The board should devise a simple mission statement which can be put on letterheads, flyers and so on, such as LABCEC's mission statement:

'To struggle for the rights of children in Laborie'.

26. Government role

See paper on Government role in Appendix 12. This should be discussed with board members, parents, sponsors and friends.

27. Constitution

See LABCEC's constitution for example of the constitution of a community education centre. See National Association's constitution for example of a network constitution.

List of Agenda topics by frequency of recurrence

Topics for every meeting	Topics for once a year	Occasional topics
1. Minutes	8. Parent educators minutes	23. Parents as teachers programme
2. Errors and omissions	9. Friends and AGM	24. Relations with other pre-schools and daycares in the area
3. Matters arising	10. Absent board members	25. Mission statement
4. Board education	11. Board turnover	26. Government role
5. Board policies	12. Scholarships	27. Constitution
6. Follow up	13. Elections	
7. AOB	14. Brainstorming for proposals out (needs of centre)	
	15. Report on annual staff evaluations	
	16. Report on annual children's evaluations	
	17. Report on self study	
	18. Annual report	
	19. Auditor's report	
	20. Report on policy monitoring	
	21. Parents on board	
	22. Report on common entrance results	

Chapter 6

Local fund-raising in Early Childhood Education centres

In Saint Lucia, as in all English speaking Caribbean countries except Grenada, Government devotes very little of its budget to early childhood education. Most of the early childhood education centres must find 95% or more of their recurrent budgets. In many centres not all teachers receive their salaries for all the months of the year. What is the situation of your centre? Moreover, the salaries remain low. What are the salaries in your centre? What would you like them to be?

If most early childhood development centres can only manage to pay low salaries to trained teachers and not for all the months of the year, the situation as to meeting their other basic needs can only be imagined. For instance, do you have running water? Do you have flush toilets? Do you spend at least 10% of your annual budget on toys? Do you have a food programme? Do you have a fridge? A stove? A freezer? Do you offer full scholarships? How many per year? Do you offer partial scholarships for the poor? How many per year? What is the turnover rate of your staff?

If the amount per child for quality care in Saint Lucia was calculated in rural and urban communities, it would be seen that the cost for care far supersedes the amount given, since most centres depend for 90% or more on parent fees. Let us now calculate the amount of running expenses of your centre and compare it with your income.

MONTHLY BUDGET, 1995-1996

Month beginning .... Ending ....

ITEMS	RECEIVED/SPENT THIS MONTH	IN/OUT SEPTEMBER TO ENDING MONTH	MONTHLY TARGET
1. FUNDRAISING			
Raffle			
Photocopies			
Sponsors			
Rent			
Cake sales			
Parent meeting snacks			
Poor people's lunch			
Donors			
Other			
Other			
2. GRANTS			
3. PARENT FEES			
4. Other			
TOTAL INCOME			
TELEPHONE			
ELECTRICITY			
WATER			
TRAVEL			
PER DIEM			
TRAINING			
SALARIES			
FOOD PROGRAMME			
STAMPS			
EQUIPMENT			
PREMISES			
MISCELLANEOUS			

TOTAL EXPENSES
BALANCE IN BANK BOOK   ....
Total income at beginning of the month   ....
Total expenses at the beginning of the month   ....
Balance in ledger book (not in bank book)   ....

As you can see, your expenses far outweigh your income. If the parents cannot meet your expenses, what alternatives do you have in a developing nation like Saint Lucia in your quest for funding? Should government be asked to assume the costs the parents cannot afford? How then will quality be determined in terms of salaries for example? What happens to those parents who can afford to pay little or nothing at all? It is the opinion of one educator, Nimnicht, that a total government takeover would be a disaster. Do you agree? If government were to take over completely what would happen to your control? What would happen to the community's control? Do the centres meet all the rest of the costs? Should Government assume the costs of early childhood education for parents who can afford to pay little or nothing? Should Government assist centres only where there is evidence that the centre is doing a certain amount of fund-raising itself?

Taking all these questions into consideration, and bearing in mind quality costs in terms of teachers' salaries and replacing regular equipment, what percentage of your full quality cost can you meet with active fund-raising? Fill in the following table, bearing in mind the maximum you think you can achieve from an active fund-raising drive.

Fund-raising activities 95-96

Month ....

Activity	Persons responsible	Monthly Amount to be raised	Actually raised
1. Sponsors			
2. Cecs			
3. Cake sales			
4. Lunches			
5. Raffle			
6. Overseas grant			
7. Parent meeting snacks			
8. Rotaract Annual Bazaar			
9. Annual poor people's lunch			
10. Saturdays sales (1 or 2 per month)			
11. Meals on wheels			
12. Donors			
13. Computer Certificates			
14. Corsages			
15. Popcorn day			
16. House to house sale			
17. Icecles			
18. Icecream sales			
19. Confectionery tray			
20. Hotdogs			
21. Other			
22. Other			
23. Other			
24. Other			
Total			

Now go back to the previous table and fill in the income you think you could manage to fund-raise and balance it with the expenses you would like to be able to meet. This time do not put in the salaries you actually have but the salaries you would like to have. Remember to pay your trained teachers adequately. And to cut costs and increase community commitment and increase commitment to the poor, be sure to include volunteers, possibly receiving tiny stipends, among your adult/ child ratios.

MONTHLY BUDGET, 1995-1996

Month beginning .... Ending ....

ITEMS	RECEIVED/SPENT THIS MONTH	IN/OUT SEPTEMBER TO ENDING MONTH	MONTHLY TARGET
1. FUNDRAISING			
Raffle.			
Photocopies			
Sponsors			
Rent			
Cake sales			
Parent meeting snacks			
Poor people's lunch			
Donors			
Other			
Other			
2. GRANTS			
3. PARENT FEES			
4. Other			
TOTAL INCOME			
TELEPHONE			
ELECTRICITY			
WATER			
TRAVEL			
PER DIEM			
TRAINING			
SALARIES			
FOOD PROGRAM			
STAMPS			
EQUIPMENT			
PREMISES			
NATIONAL INSURANCE			
MISCELLANEOUS			

TOTAL EXPENSES
BALANCE IN BANK BOOK ....
Total income at beginning of the month ....
Total expenses at the beginning of the month ....
Balance in ledger book (not in bank book) ....

It is clear that even with full fund-raising drives, centres can meet no more than 70% of the amount needed for quality provision. How much did your centre reach? Should Government then assist in the impetus for community control and ownership by giving centres subventions based on the amounts they fund-raise, remembering those children who do not attend early childhood education centres and who receive inadequate parenting and who can afford to pay little or nothing? What do professionals have to say? What do parents have to say? What do Government officials have to say? What does business have to say? What do other community members have to say? Show them this paper and ask them. Keep a list of all those with whom you have discussed this paper in detail.

LABCEC is a living example that an early childhood education centre can match parent fees from recurrent local and overseas funding. But where does the balance come from to achieve minimum quality?

The types of fund-raising that your centre can do may be the traditional ones known to have worked, plus one or two new activities thrown in. The difference is that these activities should be done systematically with an education component included, stating why fund-raising for early childhood education should be a priority for all Saint Lucians.

Activities include raffles. Several communities could combine to make the prizes more attractive and having a winner from each community. Activities also include icecream sales, cake sales, lunches, donors who give small sums, donors both local and foreign who give fixed and larger sums, making corsages, traditional house to house sales such as coconut cakes, popcorn days, setting up a small confectionery or other store, sale of icecles.

However, regularity is the key to successful fund-raising. It is not one cake sale per year but eight or ten, and so on.

A fundraising organiser, starting with a small honorarium and going up, should be employed. This person could be a trained teacher, who teaches one hour a day and is assisted by volunteers when spending the rest of the day fund-raising.

All members of staff need to be involved in community fund-raising. It needs to be written into their job description. Some members, notably the administrative staff, should raise larger amounts. Yet smaller contributions need not mean that less work was involved. The centres need to ensure that there is at least one person on the staff who has reached a level of proficiency in CXC English and Math for communication skills both written and oral, as well as proficiency in financial management. It is important to understand that only those staff who have the high levels of initiative, follow-up skills and sense of community commitment, all so essential, will be able to achieve greater amounts in fund-raising.

The support of the community is vital in fund-raising. Community members are the ones who donate, who sell raffle tickets, who allow ice-cream sales and popcorn sales to be held on school premises. They buy cakes, attend the lunches and buy corsages. Children in the community buy the icicles, the icecream and the confectionery. Most important, key community members and friends can diminish criticism of the centre. What has repeatedly surfaced during fund-raising drives is criticism of the unquenchable needs of centres for financial gain. If the community truly understood the priority need for quality early childhood education, community members would not say this. Only community education on the prime importance of early childhood education and the financial needs of such a programme can limit or quench the criticism. The board members and friends of the centre are key persons in this community education, since word of mouth still remains, in rural Saint Lucia at least, the best form of communication. Pamphlets and telephone calls to key persons can help. A thorough discussion of this paper with key persons can also help.

On a positive note, early childhood education centres which invest in community fund-raising as a major means of achieving quality translate to the community in countless little way their undying love and support for Saint Lucia's children.

Note to facilitator

1. Write minutes of training session.

2. Write down answers for each question asked on manual on separate paper from minutes.

3. Keep a copy of the centre's real expenditure.

4. Keep a copy of the centre's desired expenditure.

5. Keep a copy of the list of fund-raising activities and amounts to be raised per centre.

Community fund-raising through Local Personal Donors (LPD)

All early childhood education centres need to fund-raise to meet their current budgets. This paper outlines one method of fund-raising by community based early childhood education centres through reliance on local personal donors.

Fund-raising through local personal donors on a systematic basis started at the Laborie Community Education Centre (LABCEC). This method of fund-raising was suggested by a friend of LABCEC and highly supported by LABCEC's board even when I, LABCEC's Coordinator, wanted to abandon it because it was yielding so few results. Luckily this method of fund-raising was not abandoned and we proved that its lack of success was the result of a lack of systematic application and follow-up.

In fact, through this programme LABCEC raised EC$2,640.00 in 1994, EC$6,934.15 in 1995 and EC$9,898.79 in 1996. When it is considered that Laborie has a population of only 1,000, these are indeed high grants.

The great majority of parents who pay fees to early childhood education centres in Saint Lucia cannot pay the full cost for quality education. The fees paid by the parents in many cases do not cover:

– holiday salaries for the staff

– adequate salaries for many of the administrators

– basic instructional materials for the children, such as paint, paintbrushes, paper, leggoes, blocks and books

– electricity and telephone bills.

Centres thus need to fund-raise in order to help meet the costs of these items that are essential to the centre's quality. The LPD programme offers one answer to this fund-raising drive. The goals of such fund-raising are:

– to improve the quality of early childhood education in centres

– to better stand up for the rights of children.

Centres who want to do this form of fund-raising should meet with some high-powered friends of the centre and get a list of possible donors from them, then write an initial contact letter to each one. Regular follow up of this contact letter is essential.

In order to do this fund-raising properly, a centre needs a telephone at the premises. The centre also needs, through the National Association of Early Childhood Educators, easy access to a computer, printer and fax machine.

I will now turn to an implementation plan of this form of fund-raising.

The Administrators should first call a meeting of influential friends of the centre by writing a letter to these friends. The letter should state the importance of quality early childhood education to the development of children's minds and stress that quality early childhood education is essential if Saint Lucia is to develop a nation of creative problem solvers. Quality, the letter should continue, means also community fund-raising, since parents cannot afford to pay the full cost of quality provision. Therefore, the letter should conclude, the influential friend is being asked to provide a list of possible donors to the centre.

Follow this letter with calls to the influential friends of the centre. Arrange a meeting during which the benefits of community based early childhood education centres are discussed (see NAECE for this). At this meeting and at follow-up meetings and telephone conversations, acquire a full list of names with home, office and fax numbers and full postal addresses.

Enter the names, addresses and so on on filing cards and put them in a filing box and make a list, by hand or computer, ready for the follow-up telephone calls. The list should look like this:

NAME	TELEPHONE	PROMISED TO PAY	PAID	STILL TELEPHONING
In alphabetical order	nos. home & work			

The initial contact letter to the personal donor should contain similar information to the initial letter to the influential friend.

One month after these letters are posted (ideally in June or July to coincide with the end if the centre's financial year in August) begin the follow-up telephone calls. Our experience at LABCEC has shown that one-quarter of the donors give after two to three telephone calls. Another one-quarter require many more such calls. About one-third of the donors never give at all. Do not scratch them off your list until two or three years have passed.

Donors should be sent thank you card, followed by an attractive annual report which includes a financial statement. A renewal letter of donation should be sent to each donor around July or August.

The bottom line is this:

> How committed are you to quality early childhood education?
> How much do you stand up for the rights of children?
> How comfortable are you with your centre's efforts at quality?

This task of fund-raising is the responsibility of the Administrator. If you can manage to convey to the donors your commitment, dedication and work, you are well on your way to achieving a successful Local Personal Donor programme.

Building community clusters or networks

Justification

> Centres need to get together to share human, physical, technical and financial resources

Objectives

> to build meaningful involvement of parents and wider community

> to encourage on-the-job training, a relatively inexpensive and successful form of training

to enhance the quality of the centres

to fund-raise to achieve the above objectives

Activities

- Hold parents' meetings at least twice a term.

- Hold board meetings at least once a term. The first meeting will discuss the benefits and characteristics of community based centres

- Hold Annual General Meetings once a year, including programme and financial reports as well as education

- Conduct NAECE on the job training level 1

- Hold monthly meetings of community clusters to discuss the above and other concerns. Again, the first meeting should focus on the benefits and characteristics of community based centres

- Fund-raise at minimum to run the programme and at maximum to assist the centres. This fund-raising will be based in the first instance on private and corporate donors whose names would be supplied by board members, parents and friends at the annual general meeting and in the second instance from funding agencies

Administration

Each cluster will be run by a Community Cluster Organiser (CCO) or Director. She will help in the organisation of all the activities above, be present at all parents' and board meetings initially and run the fund-raising programme. Her stipend or honourarium will be part of the administration and communication costs, ie the minimum fund-raising possible to run the programme. The CCO will participate in a three day training programme.

Evaluation

Evaluation will be integrated as a regular component at the end of each meeting by each set of stakeholders. This will be compiled into a document at the end of each year and form part of the annual report.

APPENDIX I

JOB DESCRIPTION

Administrator

Applicants must have at least CXC English and Math at Grade 3 General Proficiency. They must have three years training at the Ministry of Education, SERVOL, Trinidad or other relevant institution.

Please note that in the evaluation points 1, 2, 3, 4 or 5 can be given for the performance of each duty. Point 1 is the lowest and Point 5 the highest.

- Organise monthly parent meetings

- Keep daily activity plans

- Teach

- Keep curriculum checklists

- Evaluate children's progress yearly and send individual, assessment reports to parents

- Facilitate Christmas party and graduation exercise

- Keep account book

- Sit on the board

- Conduct and attend all training sessions required

- Attend monthly meetings of Community Development when numbers are sufficient

- Do shopping for kitchen

- Post letters

- Pay National Insurance

- Conduct transactions with Credit Union and Bank

- Pay electricity, telephone and water bills promptly

- Read at least two books per term from library. Write summaries and discuss with project advisor

- Type correspondence

- Ensure that there is a stock of receipt books

- Make the parent receipt books

- Collect parcels from post office

- Be proficient at the computer

- Prepare monthly statements

- Prepare yearly statements

- Attend meetings of the NAECE

- Sit on the board

- Liaise with Ministries concerned

- Keep monthly staff meetings and records of the same

- Be responsible for the maintainance of the centre

- Supervise all teachers and volunteers

- Ensure that the yearly evaluation is done for the 3-5's

- Ensure that the Ministry of Education's licensing requirements are met

- Receive all fees

- Publish a newsletter once per term

- Do all training for untrained staff

- Conduct parent workshops to make low cost and local materials which are culturally and racially relevant once per term

- Give to each parent an individual description of each child's intellectual, social, emotional, physical, creative and spiritual development yearly

- Conduct an annual self-study and programme evaluation

- Be proficient in the management of all financial accounts of the centre

- Management on an equal basis of the sponsorship programme

- Management on an equal basis of the local fund-raising and income generation programme

- Keep book for recording accidents and book for recording children's medical problems

- Conduct annual parent evaluations

- Organise classroom volunteers and substitutes

APPENDIX 2

PARENT EDUCATORS

AGENDA PARENT EDUCATORS MEETING;
COMMENTS ON PARENT EDUCATORS' MINUTES
(as at LABCEC TUESDAY, MAY 24TH, 1994 5.00 P.M.)

1. List of parents visited last year, children and parent educators

2. List of parents visited this year, children and parent educators

3. Presentations to government district representatives.

4. Sancha. parent in overcrowded house. Investigate further. Write report

5. Committee to prepare report to budget committee of ministry of education and culture. Discuss topics

6. Presentations to friends

7. Comments on Minutes

8. AOB importance of filling out questionnaires well (used to evaluate work done by parent educator)

9. Date and time of next meeting (two months hence)

(Please note that all names are fictional)

Sancha Helly
Sancha did not include expense accounts. Please do so next time. Sancha interviewed a parent who recognised clearly the importance of the programme and her own mistakes as a parent. The parent said 'This programme has helped my daughter with medical treatment and a low cost of pre-school. Now Mrs. Donata and another lady is trying to assist me. All of this started during the home visit programme although I have not helped my kids as I should'. Evidently, the parent is feeling guilty. Sancha should recognise this guilt but not encourage it as guilt is often followed by resentment to the Parent Educator and, worse, to the children. Sancha should, rather, encourage the parent to turn over a new leaf.

Lydia Dely

Lydia wrote very good and informed minutes. However, she made a major mistake. She gave the same lesson regardless of the age of the child. This is wrong. Lydia should not repeat this mistake. Lydia said that when she arrived at Myrtle Singh's home, she found Myrtle and one of the fathers quarrelling, cursing and all. Sandra should try her best to discourage such behaviour. Lydia mentioned that Myrtle is addicted to smoking and this was the reason for a premature baby weighing only two pounds. Is this true? If so, what can be done? Can the parent be referred for example? Worse still, Myrtle also noted that the nurses told her if she had another child she would die. Is this true? Can this be checked by a doctor? Lydia should do follow-up on the parent Fellicia who took one of the children's father to social welfare for child support and is taking him to court. Lydia noted that Fostin's child's father is a drug addict and smokes a lot. This is not the only case Lydia mentions of drug addiction. What can we do? The problems seem many. Of Antonia, Lydia noted that they all lived together in a small house which is inadequate to accommodate so many people. When she got there, she found all of them naked and Antonia was sharing food on the floor. Should a scholarship be given in the case of Betty Monnie? She told Lydia things were very hard and she desperately wanted and needed a job but she had no-one to take care of her child for her. Also, is a scholarship needed in the case of Marciana who cannot afford to send her children to school every day. Annselma shouts at her children a lot. Lydia talked to her about it. This was good. She should continue to do so.

Lydia should fill in all the lines of her family information form, even if she puts in a blank for employment, for example. Lydia should, at least for one minute, describe each separate lesson she gives in detail. Lydia noted that Rosamunde is a diabetic and is also suffering from sickle-cell anaemia. Rosamunde was very positive about the programme. She said she never knew she had to teach and observe such things at an early age. Can we help Rosamunde? Again another case of a grandmother being very positive. She commended the programme and said that it was very interesting. Dannie only speaks creole to her children. We have talked about how to approach this already. What did we say? Dannie's child's father uses a lot of obscene language to his children. How can we counter this? Vereba also seems to need a scholarship. She said that her first daughter was attending pre-school and because of financial problems she had to remove her from school. Also Henrietta's son was recently attending the Happy House Pre-School but because of financial problems he had to stop. One parent, Josephina, was so impressed with the programme that she said she was willing to send her child to school next month. Has she done so?

Daniel Orphalina

Daniel seems to have a problem relating to her understanding of child development. She noted of a three year old that the child 'misbehaves very much'. One cannot talk of a three year old misbehaving. The child may be very active but she is not in enough control of her actions to be deemed misbehaving. Again, Daniel writes 'The problem is that the child doesn't listen to me'. Why should the child listen to you, Daniel? She is only learning to listen. Prala's mother noted that Michael is getting better each time and he is good with numbers. This is good. Daniel calls Gan Arthury a problem child. Can she explain?

Dara White

Dara, why did you do two visits per month? Please only do one visit per month. But maybe you have an explanation. Dara made a very good remark when she said, 'I try my best with him. He has very little patience and you must know how to work with him', when talking of Edwina's child. This shows good flexibility on Dara's part. This same child's mother said he was developing his fine muscles. Good. Dara seems to have very good rapport with her children. She noted Sira was very happy when she saw her.

Moody Sim

Alexandrina is developing under Moody's guidance. Moody noted the parent as saying that the topics have made her see herself as abusive sometimes, especially in her criticism of mistakes and calling her children names and beating them. The parent went on to say that the programme has been of help to her and she took time to read out the handouts left over and over again. Again another evidence of self-awareness in Moody's parents. Adelina noted that she was guilty of all in the list of the ways parents can discourage their children's self-esteem. Moody noted that Joelina Smity bought books for her child. Good. She noted that Anne Yarde still had an eye problem. What can be done? What has been done? Can we find the medicine prescribed by Dr. Arthur which cannot be found in Saint Lucia? Moody explained to a parent why primary colours are called such. Do all home visitors know this? Can Moody explain? Again, a parent improves. Mora Doonstick noted that she did most things on the discouraging list and says she will try not to do them.

Ann Alexander

Ann gave a most touching rendition of a child's trust in her. When he reached Khrishna's residence, he came close to her and said 'I love you'. Khrishna's mother said that a workshop should be organised to show parents how to make simple toys for their children. Huntelina says she has seen a huge improvement in her son since the advent of the programme. Huntelina noted that one form of punishment she received from her parents was that she was left without food. It is important to stress that food is a basic need and on no account should withdrawal of basic needs be used as a form of punishment. Ann noted that baby Kumina laughed and screamed. Exciting. Ann noted that Lucy and Dave Edwards once again congratulated the programme and said it should go on forever. Ann gave these parents some activities to do with their child. This is very praiseworthy.

APPENDIX 3

APPEAL FOR FUNDS
(Sample letter as sent by LABCEC)

The Laborie Community Education Centre
LABCEC
Laborie Post Office
Saint Lucia
West Indies
Fax: 455-9194
Phone: 4546449

10th March, 1997

(Title and address of recipient)

Dear Sir or Madam,

The Laborie Community Education centre requests that you help support a child to the sum of $110.00 per year or more.

In the 21st century, Saint Lucia, like the rest of the Caribbean, will depend heavily on foreign investment for the growth of its economy.

If investors are to invest, the Saint Lucian workforce must be competitive. To do so the Saint Lucian workers must be intelligent, efficient, creative and hard workers. Gone will be the days when a country can get by with a small corps of efficient workers.

No country in the world will be able to generate full employment. Saint Lucia, as a developing country, will be able to generate even less employment than most developed countries.

Our youth and adults must be able *also* to generate self-employment. To do so, they must be creative, problem-solvers and risk takers. These skills are developed before age 8 for the most part.

Likewise, if Saint Lucia is to achieve total development for its people – socially, physically, intellectually, creatively, emotionally and spiritually, then the total development of its children is a priority need.

LABCEC's mission statement is: *To stand up for the rights of children in Laborie and its environs.*

80% of a person's brain is formed before age 8. The other 20% is formed by age 17. The total development of the child during birth – 8 is critical to St. Lucia's economic, social, political and cultural development.

The challenges to Saint Lucia during the 21st century will be gigantic. To cope with these challenges, Saint Lucian people must be flexible problem solvers, be creative and have communicative competence. These skills are acquired during the early years. The most successful university graduates have had solid foundations.

LABCEC concentrates on the child from birth to aged 5, when 50% of the brain is formed through pre-schools and Day cares and a parenting programme.

Quality early childhood education centres, like LABCEC, which concentrate on the child's total development as opposed to only academic growth, can truly make the difference between our country's going backwards or going forwards.

Finally, please note that most parents in Saint Lucia, like elsewhere in the developing Caribbean, can only afford to pay half the cost of quality early childhood education and 18% of the parents can afford to pay nothing. Without quality early childhood education (which includes a parenting programme for the 0-3 year olds) most Saint Lucian children stand little chance of grappling with the concerns of the next generation.

We do hope you will find it possible to begin to donate to LABCEC.

Yours sincerely,

Rosamunde Renard (Coordinator)

Board Members
Ulric Alphonse
Veronica Cotter
Augustine Dominique
Lucius Ellevic
Rudy John (Acting Chairperson)
Michelle Edwide (Secretary)
Virgie Joyeux
Jennifer Jn Baptiste
Agatha Jn Panel
Julitta Mathurin
Pearl Percil
Rosamunde Renard (Treasurer)
Beatrice Roland
Gilbert Wilson

APPENDIX 4

THE BANSE COMMUNITY EDUCATION CENTRE
BANCEC

5th May, 1994

Dear **FRIEND**,

It has been recognised that 80% of a child's brainpower is developed between the age of 0-6 years. As a result it is of fundamental importance that we should do all we can to help the development of Early Childhood Education Centres with active involvement of parents, to ensure the proper development of children in these early years. It is equally important that this development should be an integrated one and involve the spiritual, physical, intellectual, creative, emotional and social aspects of the child's life.

To facilitate this process, BANCEC's board is attempting to promote the growth of a voluntary organisation called **THE FRIENDS OF BANCEC**. The purpose of this organisation is to educate the local community on the importance of early childhood care and education as well as providing financial support for a high quality programme.

You are cordially invited to become a member of **FRIENDS**.

Sincerely,

....

Board Member

APPENDIX 5

NECEC
PROJECTED ANNUAL BUDGET
1994-1995

FEES EC$130.00 per term
or EC$33.00 for twelve months or EC$44 for 9 months
or EC$75.00 for six months
NUMBER OF CHILDREN 60
REGISTRATION 30.00

ITEM	REQUIRED	PARENTS	FUND-RAISE	MINISTRIES	OTHER
1. Director					
100 * 12	1,200.00	1,200.00	–	–	–
2. Head					
800*12	9,600.00	9,600.00	–	–	–
3. Teacher					
450*12	5,400.00	5,400.00	–	–	–
4. Rent	6,000.00	6,000.00	–	–	–
5. N.I.S.	918.00	918.00	–	–	–
6. G.L.I.	750.00	–	750.00	–	–
7. Materials	3,000.00	–	3,000.00	–	–
8. PAT	5,000.00	–	–	5,000.00	–
9.Teacher					
280*12	3,360.00	–	3,360.00	–	–
10. Post	400.00	–	400.00	–	–
11.Admin/Commun.	800.00	–	800.00	–	–
12.Travel	400.00	–	400.00	–	–
13.Contigencies	1,200.00	–	1,200.00	–	–
TOTALS	38,028.00	22,200.00	10,828.00	5,000.00	–

APPENDIX 6

PARENTS' GROUP MEETINGS

TOPICS

RESOURCE PERSON CHOICE	TOPIC COMMUNITY
1. Principal of Infant or Combined	What the Infant School expects of the incoming Pre-School child
2. Local Nurse	Immunisation and other health matters
3. Lawyer	Legal matters pertaining to children
4. Community Development	Fathers paying Child Support or Social Services
5. Resource Person	Child Abuse
6. Resource Person	Discipline: Alternatives to corporal punishment
7. Pre-School Administrator	The importance of play and toys in child's learning
8. Parent Educators	Exposé on the Parenting Programme with skit
9. Teacher/Librarian	The importance of reading and storybooks in children's learning
10. Bank Manager	Loans available to the public and requirements
11. Math Teacher	Math games to teach your child for a secure foundation in number
12. Nutrition specialist	Good nutrition for your children
13. Diet specialist	Diet and your health with Pre-School Administrator as resource person
14. Exercise Resource person	Exercise and your health
15. Local Musician	Play musical instrument for 10-15 minutes. Speaker to introduce musician and his/her contribution to the community
16. Panel of old community notables	The community long ago
17. Panel of Youth	The community as we see it at present
18. Environmentalist	How community members can help protect the environment

19. Panel of prominent community representatives (District rep, Priest)	The Community as we see it at present. Projections for the future
20.	Same panel as above with different people
21. Board members	The significance of the Pre-School board and my role on it.
22. Hotelier	How my hotel can interact with the community in order to help it
23. Resource Person	The attributes of a quality Pre-School and DayCare and how this centre plans to achieve it.
24. Resource Person	Child Abuse and Individual Counselling
25. Resource Person	General Liability Insurance
26. Resource Person	Skills of communication with other people
27. Resource Person	Family relationships
28. Resource Person	Puberty and introducing sex education to the 9-10 year old child
29. Teacher 2 per	Curriculum – Language Arts, Math, Art, Concept Formation (done 1 or year for four years and then repeated)
30. Administrator	Written policies
31. Resource Person	Mission Statement
32.	Creating a safe environment for children
33.	Establishing healthy sleep patterns
34.	Building self-esteem
35.	Understanding and encouraging Language Development
36.	Reading aloud – effective ways to use books
37.	Play activities for parents and children together
38.	Book and toy-making
39.	Sibling rivalry
40.	Toilet teaching
41.	Understanding parent stress and child stress
42.	Rules and regulations of the school and the classroom
43.	Specific tasks of parent volunteers, how to perform them, and any necessary special preparations, limits of responsibilities and duties
44.	Classroom management techniques
45.	A survey of parent interests and abilities
47.	See two books *Pathways to Parenting,* produced by Parenting Partners, Jamaica
48.	See the National Association of Early Childhood Educators, Saint Lucia, training Level 1 for additional material.

APPENDIX 7

STAFF QUESTIONNAIRE

Staff Children Interaction

		Not at all	Sometimes	Very much

1.1   Do you smile, touch and hold the children?

1.2   Do you talk with and listen to children during worktime, structured activities, playground, when arriving and when departing?

1.3   Do you converse a lot with the children

1.4   Do you give children one to one attention when feeding, bathing or diapering them or taking them to the toilet?

1.4 a   Give examples showing any one or more of the above.

2.1   Do you quickly comfort a crying child?

2.2   Do you make crying children feel safe?

2.3   Do you listen to the children with attention and respect?

2.4   Do you respond to children's requests and questions?

2.5   Do you often look up from your group or work at the entire class?

2.6   Do you observe each child without interrupting actively involved children?

2.7 a   Give examples of any one or more of the above of the above.

	Not at all	Sometimes	Very much

3.1   Do you speak to individual children often?

3.2   Do you include children in conversations, describe things which happened, experiences you had and listen to their comments and suggestions?

3.3   Do you stoop or sit down on a low chair often so you can speak to the children at their eye level?

3.4   Do you call the children by name?

3.4 a   Give examples of any one or more of the above.

4.1   Do you talk with individual children and encourage all children to use language? For example, do you repeat the sounds of the toddlers, talk about things toddlers see, ask 2 year olds questions which make them answer in long sentences instead of just yes or no or other one word answers? Do you ask more how, why and what questions (these are open ended questions) than when and where questions?

4.2   Do you treat children of all races, religions and family backgrounds and cultures equally with respect and consideration? For example, do you see African hair also as good hair and the African nose as good as the European or the Indian – and say so to the children?

4.2 a   Give examples of any one or more of the above.

5   Do you provide children of both sexes with equal opportunities to take part in all activities? For example do you use words such as strong, gentle, pretty, helpful for both girls and boys and do you not divide into single sex groups?

Give examples of the above.

6   Do you encourage independence in children? For example, do you allow the older children to feed themselves, the toddlers to wash their hands and select their own toys, the 3 and 4 year olds to dress and pick up toys, the 4-5s to set the table, clean and help themselves?

Give examples of the above.

	Not at all	Sometimes	Very much

7   Do you use positive approaches to help the children behave constructively? For example, do you change the subject when a child is upset, plan, praise children for good behaviour, discuss the rules of the class with the children, describe situations rather than give your own solutions?

Give examples of the above.

8   Do you refrain from using physical punishment, calling children names or frightening the children and making them feel ashamed?

Give examples of the above.

9   Do you help children to deal with anger, sadness and frustration by comforting, identifying, reflecting feelings and helping children use words to solve their problems?

Give examples of the above.

10   Do you encourage pro-social behaviours in children such as cooperating, helping, taking turns and talking to solve problems? For example, do you role-model good behaviours, do you search for ways to develop pro-social behaviours and describe them? Do you initiate opportunities for exploring and valuing differences?

Give examples of the above.

11   Do you encourage children to talk about feelings and ideas instead of using force? For example, do you supply appropriate words for infants and toddlers to help them learn ways to get along in a group? Do you step in quickly when children start fighting and discuss with them why fighting is inappropriate? Do you discuss other solutions children could take with 2 year olds and older?

Give examples of the above.

12.1   Do you read to at least one child per day?

12.2   Do you count with at least one child per day using beans, matches or whatever is available?

12.3   Do you take good care of the toys so that the supply provided does not quickly diminish?

Give examples of the above.

Health, Safety and Nutrition

		Not at all	Sometimes	Very much

1.1   Do you see that tables are washed and floors are swept after meals?

1.2   Do you see toys are picked up after use?

2.1   For Daycare only: Do you ensure that soiled diapers are put in closed rubbish bin and that soiled clothes are kept in a closed container out of reach of the children?

2.2   Do you regularly help keep the toilet area clean?

3   Do you clean the water-play containers daily with chemico?

4   Do you see that drinking water is always available for the children within their reach?

5   Do you see children wash hands after going to the toilet and before meals?

6   Do you encourage the children to assist with cleaning up after meals?

7   Do you sit with the children and converse with them regularly during snack and lunch time?

Staff Parent Interaction

1   Do you keep a daily diary of important happenings to the children, good and bad, so you can inform parents?

2   Do you attend six (6) parent meetings per year?

3   For teachers-in-charge only: Do you inform parents about important matters or about changes taking place at your centre, through newsletters, bulletin boards, frequent notes, telephone calls and so on?

4   When a parent brings a complaint and/or other matter to your attention, do you listen to the parent, state your agreement first with the points you agree with and only afterwards mention aspects that you may not necessarily agree with?

5   Do you refrain from bad-mouthing parents who bring complaints but instead discuss only the content and importance of the complaint itself?

APPENDIX 8

ADMINISTRATOR'S REPORT/CURRICULUM

		Not at all	Sometimes	Very much

I   The programme has written policies and the centre's mission statement and objectives is available to all staff and parents. This policy covers hours, fees, illness, holidays, refund information and termination of enrolment

2.1   The programmeme has a written curriculum based on up-to-date knowledge of child development

2.2   Activity plans are regularly done and kept available for Administrator and parents

2.3   The learning environment and activities for children reflect the programme's philosophy and goals

3.1   Adaptations are made in the environment and staffing patterns for children with special needs

3.2   Staff refer children to appropriate professionals when necessary

3.3   When disabled, developmentally delayed or emotionally disturbed children are cared for, staff are aware of the identified/ diagnosed special needs of each child and are trained to follow through on specific intervention plans

3.4   Parents are involved in development and use of individual education plans for children with special needs. Staff address the needs of parents of children with special needs

4.1   There is a written timetable for each group of children

4.2   All age groups play outdoors daily, weather permitting

4.3   The timetable provides for periods of both quiet and active play

4.4   There are at least five different learning areas in each classroom

4.5   Children aged under $2^1/_2$ years are not expected to function as a large group

	Not at all	Sometimes	Very much

4.6 A balance of large muscle/small muscle activities is provided

4.7 There is a time each day when children initiate activities and a time when staff initiate activities.

ADMINISTRATOR'S REPORT – STAFFING

	Not at all	Sometimes	Very much

1.1 There should be 1 adult to 3-4 infants

1.2 There should be 1 adult per 5-6 children aged under $2^1/_2$ years

2 There should be 1 adult for 10-12 children from $2^1/_2$-5 years

3 Substitutes are provided to maintain staff-child ratios when regular staff are absent

4.1 Every attempt is made to have continuity of adults who work with children

4.2 Infants and toddlers spend majority of the time interacting with the same person each day

4.3 There should be a minimum of 25-35 square feet of usable classroom space per child indoors

4.4 There should be a minimum of 75 square feet per child of play space outdoors

5 Records are kept of staff's résumé, on the job training and results of evaluations

6 The centre has written policies defining the role and responsibilities of board members and staff

7 Board Members and Principals of the Infant and Primary Schools are informed of the elements and methods involved in developing a high quality programme

8 Minutes of Board Meetings are kept

9 Financial accounts are kept

10 Accident protection and liability insurance is maintained for children and adults (Government regulations)

11 The Administrator uses the community resources available, including Health Aides, food producers and so on

12 Staff and Administrator communicate frequently about the programme, children and families

		Not at all	Sometimes	Very much
12.1	Staff plan and consult together			
12.2	Regular staff meetings are held			
12.3	Staff are allocated paid planning time			
13.1	Staff are allowed breaks of at least 15 minutes for each 4 hour period			
13.2	Staff keep information confidential about children, families and other staff members. They do not comment about children or parents in presence of other adults or children			
13.3	An appropriate person-on-site is designated to assume authority and take action in the event of Director's absence			
14	The programme meets the licensing requirements of the Ministry of Education.			

ADMINISTRATOR'S REPORT – ADMINISTRATION

		Not at all	Sometimes	Very much
1	At least annually, the Administrator and staff conduct a self-study looking at self-children interaction, staff-parent interaction, health, safety and nutrition, the Administrator's reports, activity plans, training reports, classroom observations, staff duties assigned and staff conduct of their job description			
2	The centre has written personnel policies including job descriptions, compensation with increments based in performance and training, resignation and termination benefits and grievance procedures			
3	Benefits packages for full time staff members include paid leave (annual, sick and personal), NIS benefits, subsidised daycare and pre-school for their own children. Educational benefits should be the same for volunteers			
4	Attendance records of staff and children are kept			

ADMINISTRATOR'S REPORT

Staff Qualifications and Development

	Not at all	Sometimes	Very much

1.1 Teachers-in-charge are 18 years of age or older. Volunteers are 16 years of age and older, receive orientation and only work with children under supervision of trained staff members.

1.2 All teachers and volunteers participate in regular on the job training by the Ministry, NAECE or other relevant institutions

1.3 Teachers in charge have completed or are in the process of completing the Ministry's one year training programme or NAECE's Level 2 training programme

2.1 The Administrator has completed or is completing the Ministry's one year training programme or NAECE's Level 2 training programme

2.2 New staff are adequately oriented about the goals and philosophy of the programme, emergency health and safety procedures, special needs of children assigned to the staff member's care, guidance and classroom management techniques, planned daily activities of the programme, and expectations for ethical conduct.

3.1 Accurate and current records are kept of staff qualifications.

The self-study of the National Association for the Education of Young Children (NAEYCE) was a source of inspiration for the above.

APPENDIX 10

LICENSING REQUIREMENTS
(Summary)

Write a letter requesting registration of pre-school and requesting application forms and a list of supporting documents required for completion of an application for license (application form to be submitted within 3 months)

FORMS

1. Fire Department inspection and approval

2. Ministry of Health inspection and approval

3. Central Planning Unit inspection and approval

4. General liability insurance

5. Projected annual budget

6. Certificate of incorporation

7. Medical examinations for staff and children

8. Timetables

9. Curriculum

10. Menus

11. Evacuation

12. Parenting – Home Visits

13. Parenting – Group Meetings

14. Parenting – Open Days

15. Parenting – Newsletter

16. Job Descriptions

17. Staff references

18. Staff child ratio for each group

19. Training evidence

20. Application forms

21. Diagrammatic floor plan (25 square feet per child)

PHYSICAL PLANT

1. Children's garments separately hung up
2. Separate staff toilet
3. Adequate office space
4. 4 year olds in separate area
5. Adequate light and ventilation
6. One cot per child
7. 1 toilet per 10 children
8. Outdoor space
9. Area for sick children
10. Centre kept clean
11. Adequate water facilities
12. Sewage and pit facilities
13. Concrete floors covered
14. Garbage receptacles covered and not stored in same room with children, except for paper
15. Individual drinking cups
16. No sharing of washcloths, toothbrushes, towels, combs, hairbrushes
17. Fire extinguisher
18. Stairs, walkways, ramps and porches free from accumulation of water
19. Written plan for emergency evacuation
20. Fire drills once a month. Records kept
21. Lead free paint
22. First Aid kit adequately stocked
23. Flammable liquids etc. inaccessible to children
24. Covers for electrical outlets
25. Telephone numbers for fire, police, medical assistance posted on telephone book

Programme

1. Corporal punishment and humiliating or frightening methods of control or discipline shall be prohibited
2. Punishment shall *not be* associated with food, rest, toilet training, isolation
3. A registered nurse shall visit the centre at least once a week (under supervision)

RECORDS

1. Name, address, sex, date of birth of each child
2. Where parents and guardians can be reached in case of emergency
3. Names and addresses to which children can be released
4. Daily attendance records
5. Health cards
6. Child and staff health examinations

OTHER

1.   Cribs or cots should be situated at least 2 feet apart

2.   No pillows

3.   Toilet equipment such as potties

4.   Children taken outdoors every day except when raining

5.   Children not left without supervision at any time

6.   Only person 18 years of age or secondary school graduate shall be left in full charge of children at any time

STAFFING

1.   All staff shall have physical examination by a physician prior to employment and annually thereafter with tuberculin tests or chest X-rays

2.   No person on duty should have respiratory, gastro-intestinal or skin infection or other communicable diseases

3.   Group leaders working with children of age 3 or under should have specific experience or training in infant/toddler care

APPENDIX 10

WRITTEN POLICIES

LABORIE PRE-SCHOOL AND DAYCARE
'LABCEC'
1994

The Laborie Community Education Centre's policies are to cater for the total development of the child, through the SPICES curriculum. SPICES is as follows:

1. **Social Development**
Children have to get along with others in the home, at school and in the community. To practice social graces and to have social interaction with others.

2. **Physical Development**
Children will have opportunities to develop their large and small muscles.

3. **Intellectual Development**
Children have to gain knowledge to think, to communicate and to solve problems in all areas of the curriculum.

4. **Creative Development**
Children will be given the opportunity to use their imagination to create ideas and express themselves in areas of music, craft, drama and visual arts.

5. **Emotional Development**
Children will learn to develop their self-confidence, self-esteem and self-awareness and to express their feelings in a positive way.

6. **Spiritual Development**
Children need to learn moral values. They will learn how to appreciate and love others and the world around them.

RULES OF LABCEC

1. LABCEC is a not-for-profit pre-school and daycare or early childhood education centre with a continuing education programme in the form of a parents as teachers programme and a CXC programme

2. The hours of operation of its pre-school are from 7.30am to 3pm

3. The hours of operation of its daycare are from 7.30am to 4.30pm

4. One morning snack and one lunch per day are served

5. Children are admitted from the age of 1 year up to the age of 5 years

6. Parents must provide health cards with all the relevant vaccines on registration. Parents must fill out all the sections of the registration forms including the section on ailments of child

7. The maximum number of children to be admitted to the Laborie pre-school and daycare is 95.

8. There are four levels of fees:
    1. EC$220.00 per term. Parents may pay this in three months at EC$75.00 per month or in four months at EC$60.00 per month. This fee includes one lunch and one snack per day.

    2. EC$146.00 per term. Parents may pay this in three months at EC$48.00 per month or in four months at EC$36.00 per month. This fee does not include lunch but includes one snack.

    3. EC$146.00 per term. Parents may pay this in three months at EC$48.00 per month or in four months at EC$36.00 per month. This fee is for children between the ages of 1-2 years including full food programme.

    4. EC$110.00 per term. Paarents may pay this in three months at EC$37.00 per month or in four months at EC$28.00 per month. This fee does not include food programme although underprivileged children may apply to have their children included in the food programme

9. Any parent who can afford to pay only EC$10.00 or less per month for their child's early childhood education including food programmeshould apply to LABCEC's board for a scholarship. Parents and board members should recommend such persons. These children would be entitled to participate in the food programme

10. Any child who is absent for a month or more is exempted from paying school fees

11. In case of disaster warnings children should be kept home – eg. heavy rains, storms, hurricanes

12. Children who are affected by contagious diseases should be kept away from school to avoid the spread of the disease, and a doctor's certificate should be presented on their return

13. Parents are requested to attend meetings once per month

14. A cup should be provided for your child (children should not use one another's utensils)

15. School fees must be paid by the first week of every month. If you fail to do so, without an excuse, your child will be sent back home.

16. There is an initial registration fee of EC$30.00, payable once only.

17. An extra set of clothing should be included in the child's bag and a plastic bag for any wet or soiled clothes.

18. Parents should label children's belongings such as: bags, caps, raincoats, umbrellas and lunch kits.

19. Children in the daycare should bring with them their own:

> towel
> comb
> brush
> bottle
> change of clothes

20. Parents are requested to sign a special permission form for their children to attend field trips, in addition to the permission they give on the registration forms

21. If we have excluded any requirements which you think should form part of these written policies please do not hesitate to inform us. Please note that personnel policies including job descriptions, pay ranges, benefits and NIS will be treated separately.

APPENDIX 11

PERSONNEL POLICY

THE LABORIE COMMUNITY EDUCATION CENTRE

Citrus Grove,
Laborie,
Saint Lucia,
West Indies

A. SALARIES

Salaries are to be set for each employee according to agreement between the employee, the Coordinator and the other Administrative staff, subject to the approval of the Board of Directors. Salaries will be based on abilities, training, length of service, education, experience and job responsibilities. Payment will be made on the last day of each month or on the working day that falls closest. Salary increases shall be commensurate with increased enrolment, income, duties and responsibilities of any employee.

B. VACATION PAY

No deductions from pay will be made for regular school vacations and holiday closings. Each employee should check their job description for holidays.

C. SICK OR PERSONAL LEAVE

One day a month personal leave and two days a month sick leave shall be allowed with full pay. In case of a major illness that requires an absence of more than three days, the cost of hiring a substitute shall be deducted from regular pay. After thirty school days, pay shall be terminated. Leave shall not be cumulative from year to year. Maternity leave shall be for a period not exceeding three months and without pay but NIS will give maternity benefits. Note that NIS also pays 65% of worker's insurable earnings for a period of illness in excess of three days and the employer pays 35% for sick and maternity leave as per NIS rules.

D. SUBSTITUTES OR SUPPLY TEACHERS

Substitutes hired by the Coordinator upon the absence of a teacher shall be paid according to the rate provided in the annual budget. The Headteacher is responsible for hiring them or, in her absence, the Deputy Headteacher.

E. **HOURS**

Teachers shall work from four to eight hours daily, depending upon individual contracts. Teachers are expected to attend staff meetings of one-half to two hours weekly. Time for such meetings and for classroom preparation is built into the salary schedule. All salaried persons may be called in for a reasonable amount of extra time at no extra pay in emergency situations, in preparation for meetings, open house or other special events and in connection with individual responsibilities of LABCEC. The Coordinator, Assistant Coordinator and Headteacher shall be on call at any time in connection with responsibilities of the position.

F. **INSURANCE BENEFITS**

All employees shall be covered by the National Insurance Scheme

G. **PROBATIONARY PERIOD**

All new employees shall serve a probationary period of 12 weeks. Thereafter the employment will be considered permanent or will be terminated. The Coordinator shall schedule regular periods of observation during the probationary period with ongoing feedback to the employee. Two weeks written notice from the school or from the teacher must be given in case of termination. Legally, no reason needs to be given if dismissal occurs during the probation period.

H. **YEARLY CONTRACT AND TERMINATION NOTICE**

All full-time staff shall operate on a yearly contract.

For employees of more than 12 weeks (taken from Section 6 of the contract of service Act. No. 14 of 1979), note that your contract may be terminated by giving

a)   One week notice if your period of continuous employment is more than twelve weeks but less than two years.

b)   Two weeks notice if your period of continuous employment is two years or more but less than five years;

c)   Six weeks notice if your period of continuous employment is more than ten years.

J. **COSTS OF TRAINING**

The centre shall make partial re-imbursement of tuition charged for Adult Education or University courses. This re-imbursement shall range from 25% to 50% of the tuition, depending on the number of staff members participating in courses concurrently, the expense of the course and the availability of funds within the budget. Tuition shall be paid in the form of a loan to the employee. During the 2nd year of continued employment after the completion of the course, the loan shall be written off as an expense. Should the person voluntarily leave the school's employment prior to a one year period, the amount loaned will be deducted from the person's final paycheck.

Travel and per diem for all courses will be paid by the centre unless the organising body of the training course pays a per diem and travel costs.

L. All staff persons shall have a fifteen minute relief period in every four hours of work. Adequate supervision of the students will be arranged.

M. **HEALTH EXAMINATION**

See licensing requirements

N. **SUPERVISION**

The staff will be responsible to the Headteacher of the Centre. In the Headteacher's absence, the staff will be responsible to the Deputy Headteacher. The Headteacher is responsible to the Coordinator, who is responsible to the Board of Directors.

O. **JOB DESCRIPTION**

Each member of staff shall be given a job description that will be applicable to the position covered by the contract.

P. **CONTRACTS**

Each staff member will be given a yearly contract

Q. **PERSONNEL DIFFERENCES**

In the event of lack of agreement on procedure between members of the teaching staff, the Coordinator will make the final decision. In the event of lack of agreement on procedure between members of the teaching staff and the Coordinator, the Coordinator may ask the Chairperson of the Board to arbitrate and will abide by the Chairperson's decision.

R. **STAFFING**

The administrative team is responsible for staffing and for hiring and firing staff. Staff members who feel they have been unfairly dismissed may appeal to the board.

S. **AMENDMENTS**

Any changes, revisions, or amendments to the personnel policy will be presented to each staff member at least ten days before the offering of a new contract.

EMPLOYMENT AGREEMENT FORM

THE LABORIE COMMUNITY EDUCATION CENTRE AND ...

Dear.............. ,

You are invited to become/continue as a member of our staff for the school year beginning .... and ending ....

Your position will be that of .... with responsibilities according to your job description and the personnel policies of the school.

You will be paid at the rate of ....per month/per day.

Your hours have been set to be from no later than ....a.m. until at least ....p.m. on every day that the school is open with the exception of days on which you are on holiday, sick or personal leave.

You are expected to make yourself available for staff meetings and/or in-service training meetings, occasional evening meetings, and pertinent school events. Pay for these occasions has already been taken into consideration in setting your annual salary.

For new employees only

As a new employee, you will be on a .... month period of probation, during which time the position may be terminated by either party on giving two weeks notice.

We would like to wish you all the best during your experience at LABCEC. Welcome.

Date ....   For the Centre ....
                            Coordinator

Signature of Employee ....

Signature of Coordinator ....

THE ROLE OF GOVERNMENT IN PRE-SCHOOLS

It is clear that Early Childhood Education Centres cannot meet all their needs in their drive towards quality. The majority of parents cannot afford to budget inordinately for their child's pre-school education. So most pre-schools which are low-cost operate on shoe-string budgets. In real terms this means that Administrators of these centres earn little or no income for at least two months of the year and teachers may receive reduced income. Yet the most important part of quality is the level of training, commitment and dedication of the staff. Staff earns low salaries in most pre-schools. When, to compound this, they cannot even be sure of receiving their small incomes for all months of the year, it is easy to see why there is such a high turnover rate among Pre-School staff.

However, the needs of Pre-Schools do not only involve the provision of adequate and regular salaries. They also include such items as fences for the safety of the children, toys – which are the children's work tools – adequate housing – which sometimes implies new buildings and sometimes repaired ones – adequate water supply and electrical services. These are just some of the needs of Pre-Schools.

And yet, with all these needs, many of which are not being met presently, Pre-Schools are integral to our country's national well-being and development.

It has been proven that children's minds develop 80% during birth to 8 years. What happens to the child during these vital years is thus of vital importance to the country's social, political, economic and cultural development. Without proper attention to the years birth-8, our country's crime rate goes up, self-employment goes down, our workforce is affected negatively and extra millions of dollars are spent on solving problems which could have been prevented in the first place.

The ages of birth to 8 are, to insist, vital to our country's development. And yet, so often, they are misunderstood, ignored and underestimated. During these years, the parents, the Early Childhood Education teacher, the Infant School teacher and the wider community all play a crucial part. Efforts must be expended on their training and their well-being.

In all this, how is Government helping and how can Government help? It is not being suggested that Government should take up all the slack from the Pre-Schools. Funding agencies should play their part and so should local business. However, funding agencies will not provide salaries or any long term support, for maintenance for example. And business should reasonably be expected to assume only half the burden, at most, of this long term support.

We are not suggesting that Government take over Pre-Schools. All Pre-Schools are privately owned and we think this should continue to be the case. In developing countries such as Guyana, where Government has attempted to assume total responsibility for Early Childhood Education, the results have been problematic, according to Nimnicht*. Private management of these centres may be a necessity in these developing countries. It facilitates finance, fast decision-making and creativity in Early Childhood Education. However, Government monitoring and control is necessary to pursue a goal of achieving quality in Early Childhood Education. Government monitoring should continue to develop but along with it should develop increased responsibility towards Early Childhood Education in all domains possible.

It is in the areas of long term support which funding agencies cannot and will not supply that Government intervention is sorely needed. And undoubtedly, without this intervention, Pre-School Education for the majority of Saint Lucians will never be achieved. Government could and should help with:

1. The provision of fences for safety

2. The subvention of teachers' salaries

3. The provision of funds for building maintainance

4. The provision of start-up toys and furniture, some of which should come from local sources

5. The extension of Government training, including distance education, and follow-up already in progress

6. The provision of materials and labour costs to repair and upgrade premises

7. The identification of grant sources and support to funding agencies requesting endorsement of funding to centres and to the national association

8. The rendering of government land easily accessible and free of cost

9. Support for a National Association

These are just some of the areas in which Government could make a real contribution in the provision of quality services for pre-schools. The role of each Ministry concerned vis-a-vis points 1-9 would have to be negotiated by the Ministries and, hopefully, also by the National Association of Early Childhood Educators.

Presently, Government spends less than one percent of its budget in the Ministry of Education and the Ministry of Community Development combined, on early childhood education.

Early childhood education should be a shared responsibility between Government and community. The goal should be partnership, so that communities assume responsibility for early childhood education without being burdened with charges which are too heavy for them to bear.

So it is not being suggested that Government assume total control of Pre-Schools. This would be a mistake. Rather, that Government encourage local businesses and funding agencies to invest in Pre-School education, determine the areas where this input is not possible and then take up the slack towards the provision of quality services to Saint Lucian children and their parents.

Note

*   Glen Nimnicht *et. al.* 'Meeting the needs of young children: Policy Alternatives' (Bernard Van Leer Foundation, April 1987)